Eat, Drink and be Slim

Normal, healthy eating anytime, anywhere, every day

by Polly Hale

First published in Great Britain in 2013
Second ediłion September 2014

ISBN: 978-0-9929731-0-0

Published and designed by Shakspeare Editorial

Contents

Follow Eat Drink and be Slim

www.eatdrinkandbeslim.co.uk
www.facebook.com/EatDrinkBeSlim
www.twitter.com/eatdrinkbeslim
www.pinterest.com/pollyannahale/eat-drink-and-be-slim/
info@eatdrinkandbeslim.co.uk

Follow The Fit Mum Formula

www.thefitmumformula.com
www.facebook.com/thefitmumformula
www.twitter.com/FitMumFormula
www.pinterest.com/pollyannahale/the-fit-mum-formula/
polly@thefitmumformula.com

Buy Eat Drink and be Slim

Paperback in black and white; ebook from www.lulu.co.uk

Foreword

You have picked up this book, which probably means that a part of you, however small, is thinking about becoming healthier. What a great place to start and this book will provide you with safe, sensible and sound nutrition and lifestyle advice.

Managing body weight can seem like a battle. New 'weapons' in the war against excess weight are being churned out on a daily basis and we fight a relentless battle in our head, trying to work out what is 'good' and what is 'bad'. We are tempted with the latest fad diet, promising to dissolve inches and drop pounds in days and when we fail at these impossible and unsustainable regimes we feel like a failure. As a society we want a quick fix; we avoid taking any responsibility for our eating, hoping that the latest fad diet or slimming pill will 'sort us out' and do it for us. It won't.

We need to take back control of our relationship with food. We need to empower ourselves around food and realise that every time we put something in our mouth, we make a choice. This book is about supporting you to make the right choices.

Eating well is about balance: balancing expectations, balancing nutrients and balancing the position of food within our lives. It is not about being perfect and it is not about deprivation and hunger.

This book will guide you through the basics of eating well, not only showing you how to achieve this within the context of a busy life but also how to enjoy the journey! It is packed full of delicious recipes and genuinely useful tips that will ease you into your new healthier lifestyle.

This is a hugely valuable book. A no-nonsense approach that shows quite brilliantly that it is indeed possible to eat, drink and be slim!

Wishing you well along your healthier path and hoping that you have plenty of fun getting there.

Faith Toogood,
Bariatric Specialist Dietitian, Southmead Hospital and expert on ITV Daybreak

Acknowledgements

There are many people who have helped me put this book together, both paid and unpaid, professionals, friends and family, so firstly sorry to anyone who I forget but I expect if I know you, I will have quizzed you at some point for ideas!

Firstly to those who helped me put the book together: Gil Massara thank you for your generosity in time, help and advice, your support was so encouraging in the early days when it would have been easy to give up at every challenge. Juliet Wilson, thank you for your help with the nutritional details, I would not have had the confidence to push the book forward without you checking over it first! Richard Boult for making sure I had, grammatically speaking, not missed a thing! Thank you Aimee Byram for the advice on copyright details; another wall you helped me over. Barbara James, thanks for all the initial editing and meticulous attention to detail, for teaching me how little tweaks make the biggest of differences. Thanks H Photography for the fab cover photo, I knew you were the right choice! Thanks to Alison Shakspeare, who turned a word document into a book; tidying, reshaping and formatting it into the product you are reading, the final vital step without which this book would not exist – apart from on my laptop. Lastly, thanks so much to Faith Toogood for her warm and generous foreword as well as all the support and encouragement; you instilled confidence in my own abilities.

But mainly to my wonderful family for all the help and support. Grandma I value your opinions and feedback so thanks for reading it, and a big thanks to Lauren Cubbage for reading early versions and as a result prompting me to make huge progressions towards what the book is today. For my parents and in-laws for all the support, advice and babysitting! And to many other friends and family who's brains I picked for help and ideas.

Last but not least the three people who have supported and inspired me through all the lack-of-sleep-induced grouchiness and square eyes from excessive laptop use, but I hope you are proud of the results and that I've achieved what I set out to do; my wonderful husband James and two darling children Aurora and Bella, you are the centre of my world.

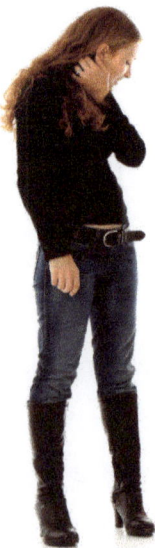

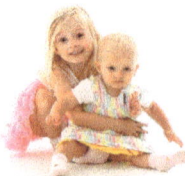

Introduction

Why I wrote this book

I wrote this book as a rebellion against the nonsense that calls itself dietary advice with which we are told every day. It's in magazines, newspapers, documentaries, TV news, and quite often our peers, family and friends who are all swapping tips on how to shed the pounds. The way the body functions is complicated – the sheer thousands of University degrees available to study would not enlighten you completely, not least for the fact that new discoveries are still being made every day which change people's perspectives on health, diet and weightloss. And the result is often another fad diet based on this 'science' while people try to capitalise on these discoveries. Hormones, genetics, lifestyle factors and the relationship between food and body chemistry all play a part, but what they all still point to is that if you eat more calories than you are burning, you will gain weight.

Despite the comments that are sometimes made to me, I am not underweight, for I am a slim but healthy BMI 20, in other words the correct weight for my height. When people call me 'skinny' I can only assume that what we have come to see as 'normal' and healthy has changed over the years – many people in the UK are at the higher end of the 'healthy' BMI range and many people are overweight, but are addressed affectionately as 'curvy', 'womanly', or 'chubby'. I have always had to be slim for either dancing or modelling, two worlds where looking good is a CV requisite, and that is how I have come to know every diet trick in the book, both healthy and unhealthy. I know how and why diets work or fail and the tricks to make losing (or gaining) weight easier. I still try and stay slim (I'm as vain as the next person) but these days by avoiding the fads and simply eating normally and healthily.

Since leaving stage school I have gained qualifications and pursued projects that have enhance my interest and knowledge in health and diet. Food and nutrition will always be a major part of my life, and in many ways that's good because we need to eat. It is fuel for our body; nothing more, nothing less. Over time food has become emotional, social, artistic, a statement of financial and social class, but at the end of the day, it is simply the fuel we need every day to keep us alive. This may sound tedious if you put it like that, so to make it more enjoyable, let's say life is too short, and we can be healthy and eat yummy food and feel satisfied. It is possible. I do it every day.

Who this book is for?

This book is written for healthy adults. It is not a 'self-help' book and I am not a counsellor. If your eating is linked to emotional or psychological issues then these may need to be addressed by an appropriately qualified professional. I am not a doctor. I can call myself a 'Nutritionist' from the training I covered during my time studying for an HND in Beauty and Health Therapy Management and with the Metabolic Effect Nutrition Consultant qualification, but not a 'Dietician' as this term requires further qualifications in dietetics and nutrition. Keep a note of this when searching for professionals in relation to diet, whether it be one-to-one consultations or the latest celebrity diet, as you don't want to be paying for the guidance of someone not much more qualified in nutrition than your average magazine editor. As with any changes to diet or exercise habits, consult your GP for advice first.

This is not even a 'diet' book. It is a re-education of normal eating that you can do anywhere, anytime, every day for the rest of your life. I won't claim it's perfect because eating the 'perfect' diet is a) difficult since there is so much conflicting information about what we should and shouldn't eat, and b) boring and at times impractical, and I want to show you how to eat without gaining weight whatever your food choices and preferences. This is normal eating.

Different metabolisms

Unfortunately our nation is becoming heavier with each year that goes by, and you only need to look at the best-seller book lists with their infinite turnover of diet books to realise many people want to lose weight. Of course we all know someone who can 'eat whatever they want' and not put on weight. Some people think that of me, but it is simply not true. Everyone has different metabolisms and what one person can happily chow down and still be skinny will make another person fat. But the fact remains that if a person consumes more calories than their body needs they will gain weight. These 'slim people' do not exceed eating what their body needs. Eating 'whatever they want' is also not the same as saying they eat every cream cake in sight. Perhaps they genuinely enjoy a healthy balanced diet, including unhealthy treats in moderation.

Did you ever watch a thin person eat? Often I have noticed they order the most fattening thing on the menu but only manage to eat a third of it. This could have something to do with fat being more filling than low fat equivalents, but is just as likely to be their appetite which they are in touch with and so stop when they are full.

A common misconception by overweight people is that they have been afflicted with a slow metabolism, that is, their body does not burn calories fast enough. Studies show that, excluding the very small percentage of people with medical reasons for a slow metabolism or difficulty losing weight (such as an underactive thyroid gland), in fact the opposite is true. The larger the person, the faster their metabolism. So an overweight person burns more calories than a slim person doing the same level of activity. This also means that the less weight you have to lose, the less you will need to eat to lose it, which is why the last few pounds are usually the hardest.

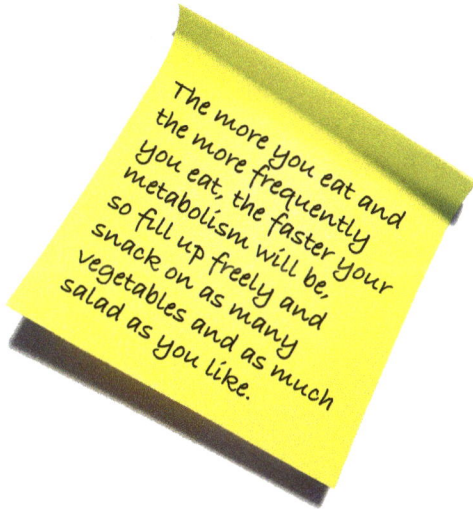

> The more you eat and the more frequently you eat, the faster your metabolism will be, so fill up freely and snack on as many vegetables and as much salad as you like.

Stop dieting and start eating

Dotted around the book you will find notes and tips to help you. If you are easily distracted you may find it helpful to put these or your own ideas or mantras around the kitchen to stop you reaching for food when you don't really want nor need it, perhaps on the fridge or cupboard doors. I've also included some of my favourite low calorie food and drink suggestions to stop you getting stuck in a rut when it comes to trying to cut down your calorie intake. You will learn as you read through this book there is no need to cut out your favourite foods, but it doesn't hurt to have a few new ideas to keep you inspired.

Years ago I once claimed that if I wrote a diet book it would contain only four words: 'Eat less, move more'. However after realising that it wasn't always as clear cut as that, I have aimed in this book to expand on that statement without changing the concept in anyway. By reading this book I do not want you to embark on another diet. Rather I want you to stop dieting, and start eating, just normally from now on! Eating should not be a battle, and foods are not 'good' or 'bad'. Eating is healthy, sociable, enjoyable and above all a necessity, so stop feeling guilty and read on . . .

1 Healthy or Slim?

This chapter looks at what it means to be slim and healthy, which are not necessarily the same thing. Whilst weight is important, how you achieve that weight, your nutritional status and your overall body composition play a big role in your overall health and fitness. The chapter also looks at some of the possible underlying reasons for weight problems and how to deal with these.

First let's look at what is health? Slim equals healthy and big is bad – right? Not necessarily. There is much, much more to health than size and weight. Some people have a tendency to store more fat around their organs such as their kidneys, liver and heart than others. They are not necessarily very overweight and often have slim limbs but have fat around their waist, meaning their vital organs are suffocating under the layers of 'internal fat', known as intra-abdominal fat and these organs can't do their jobs properly. This increases the risk of diabetes, heart disease, high blood pressure and strokes to name just a few conditions. You are more likely to be storing intra-abdominal fat if you also have a waist which measures more than 80 cm (for a woman) or 94 cm for a man.[2] This is more common in people described as an 'apple' shape. A healthy body fat percentage is considered between 10–20 percent for men and 20–30 percent for women,[3] however body fat ranges increase with age.

Body Mass Index (BMI)

BMI is a way of calculating whether your weight is in healthy proportion to your height. However it does not take into account body composition; whether your weight is a healthy balance of fat and muscle or nutritional status. The sum for calculating your BMI is:

WEIGHT (kg) divided by HEIGHT (m^2)

So for a person who is 60 kilos and stands 1.6 metres tall, the sum would be:

60 / 1.6^2 = 23.4

This person would have a healthy BMI of 23.4. BMI calculators can be found online and as phone apps which do the sums for you. Table 1 shows the range of BMIs and whether the person is underweight, obese or somewhere in between:

Under 18.5	Underweight
18.5–25	Healthy weight
25–30	Overweight
Over 30	Obese

Table 1: BMI ranges

Body Fat Percentage

Body Fat Percentage is, as the name suggests, the percentage of your body that is made up of fat. To find out your Body Fat Percentage divide your total fat by your weight. The amount of fat in your body can be measured using bio-impedance scales which work by sending a harmless electrical current (which you cannot feel) through your body and measuring the resistance as it travels through the body – muscle has a high percentage of water and conducts electricity where as fat does not and is a poor conductor. These scales are perfectly safe and your GP may have a set they can weigh you with.

So, what is healthy?

Let's look at two scenarios.

Firstly, a 45-year-old woman who smokes and likes a whisky and coke in the evening. She has a part-time job and sometimes gets up too late to eat breakfast, so she often grabs a burger on the run instead of a meal. She snacks on sweets and chocolate to keep her energy up, and if she can't be bothered to prepare something in the evening, she'll have a couple of slices of white toast with butter and marmite. She has a BMI of only 18.5, the minimum to be classed as healthy (though some professionals think 20 is a better minimum), and this makes her look much older than her years as there is no fat or muscle to fill out the contours and skin on her face and body. She never exercises apart from the ten minute walk to and from work so lacks muscle tone. Does this give you a picture of health? I think not.

Secondly, think of a 26-year-old man, a semi-professional rugby player who works as a school PE teacher. He eats three substantial but well balanced meals a day plus healthy snacks, drinks lots of water, has only a couple of beers if he's out with friends at the pub at weekends. He doesn't smoke and due to his work gets plenty of fresh air and exercise. However he has a BMI of 30 making him obese by medical standards.

Measuring a person's BMI is a really useful tool for measuring body weight: height ratios on the majority of people, but it does not indicate a person's overall nutritional health or lifestyle. BMI illustrates the need to lose or gain weight and for setting weight loss or gain goals but nothing more.

The woman does not put on weight because the total number of calories she consumes in a day do not add up to enough, even though the foods she eats are 'calorie dense' (see *Chapter 10, Feed Yourself Fuller*). She just does not eat enough of them or other foods to amount to many calories. The rugby player, though technically overweight, has a Body Fat Percentage of 10 percent (the lowest end of the recommendation for men) showing he is mostly muscle, and he is fit and healthy.

The fat gene

This title is a trick, because actually there is no fat gene, or at least none yet that aren't initially 'activated' by chronically poor nutritional intake combined with an extremely sedentary lifestyle (which probably does not apply to the majority of the population who just eat a bit too much and need to lose a few pounds). People who are overweight, have parents who are overweight and possibly also children who are overweight, have one thing in common; they all eat too much for the amount of energy they burn. How a family shops for food and eats becomes so routine that people seldom stop to think about whether anything needs to change, especially when they are rushing round the supermarket as quickly as possible during a small time-slot in their busy lives. Recipes are often handed down through generations as parents teach their children how to cook, and the foods you eat, how much and when you eat them become ingrained habits. Unfortunately as a nation each generation has become less active as we increasingly rely on machines and gadgets to do the work that would have previously been done by hand. Even in my relatively short life, the increase in use of televisions, game consoles and internet for entertainment is astounding, meaning we all spend so much more time sitting than moving around. Add to this the gradual increase in portion sizes and it's easy to see why each generation is getting fatter. Today's parents are also more likely to be working longer hours and so rely on processed and junk foods, takeaways and instant snacks such as chocolate bars, and they often don't have the energy or patience to argue or say 'no' to children who keep badgering for another biscuit.

There are, however, two hormones that influence appetite; ghrelin makes you feel hungry, while leptin tells you that you are full. Medical studies give indecisive results, but there could be a link between genetic make-up and the amounts of these two hormones that are released. For example, if one person's body releases high ghrelin levels (meaning in simple terms they become hungrier), their parents, siblings and children could also have high ghrelin levels and therefore large appetites. This does not mean that people with higher ghrelin levels store fat more easily and therefore do not put on weight easier, and having a large appetite does not mean you need more calories than other people or that you have a faster metabolism to burn calories. In the end whatever your 'natural' appetite if you consume more calories that you burn you will gain weight. (Low calorie, filling foods are required to deal with excessive hunger where calorific needs are not high; and more about these foods is written throughout the book.)

A medical condition which could be inherited is an overactive or underactive thyroid (hyperthyroidism and hypothyroidism respectively). The thyroid gland mainly produces a hormone called thyroxine, which influences the rate at which the body consumes energy from food and fat stores. Too much thyroxine and you may feel hyperactive, have trouble sleeping, sweat a lot, have an increased appetite, and lose or gain weight. Too little thyroxine and symptoms may include dry skin, depression, lethargy, hair loss and weight gain. An underactive or overactive thyroid may not need treatment if it is only mild but may require medication for more extreme cases. Both conditions are diagnosed with blood tests, so if you think you or someone in your family has a thyroid problem then contact your or their GP.

Staying healthy

How do you make sure you are slim both inside and out?

It is not just a case of being the right weight as we have shown, it's your whole lifestyle which contributes to overall wellbeing. A person's diet should be made up of mainly healthy, nutritious foods regardless of the total calories, and this should be combined with exercise. The Department of Health recommends 30 minutes exercise a day where your heart rate is slightly raised, such as brisk walking, dancing, gardening or climbing stairs. This is not as hard to achieve as you think. Buying a pedometer is one way of counting your daily steps for example. Vigorous housework or gardening also double up as useful chores that keep you fit. As an extra bonus you will not only look better by burning extra fat on the outside but being healthier on the inside will give you a sense of vitality you may have long forgotten! Smoking will inhibit your ability to get the most from your workout as it impairs lung function and reduces oxygen uptake. Alcohol not only contains a lot of calories but also inhibits nutrient absorption, decreases muscle strength and endurance and is dehydrating. People are more likely to reach for stodgy, high calorie foods after drinking as these foods line the stomach and raise sugar levels back to normal (which drop as the effects of alcohol wear off). Also, a hangover is not going to encourage you to get up and exercise! Finally here's an excuse to relax after all your hard work; a Stanford University study showed that people who had five hours or less sleep in a night had 15 percent more of the hormone ghrelin (which stimulates appetite) and 15 percent less of the hormone leptin (which lets you know you are full) than people who slept for eight hours.[4] So sleep more, and you'll want to eat less; that's got to be the best weight loss technique I ever heard!

How much to lose and how fast?

I would hazard a guess that most people want instant results. I'm afraid that aside from amputating a limb (or expensive, risky, and scar-inducing liposuction), you won't get instant results. You can, however, get results that are quicker or slower, depending on how much you cut your calorie intake and how much more exercise you take. Doctors advise aiming for a steady weight loss of around 0.5–1 kg (1–2 lb) a week, which should be easily achievable for most people when following a healthy, balanced diet, with some light exercise. For most people the higher their

BMI the faster their Basal Metabolic Rate (BMR – the rate at which they burn calories when resting) as they need the extra energy simply to 'live' and carry around the extra weight. So usually the more weight you have to lose the easier it is to do. On the other hand, people with only a small amount of weight to lose will have slower metabolisms so will find losing the weight harder, and may need to cut down further on calories or take up more exercise to achieve a goal weight.

Instead of turning to some faddy, quick fix and most importantly temporary diet, if you embark on a new way of eating, a way that you can continue for life, you will not only reach a healthy weight naturally, but you will also learn how to eat properly along the way. You can still enjoy all the foods you like with no deprivation, and you will **KEEP THE WEIGHT OFF FOR LIFE!**

However, as I said before, you can speed up the process by eating even less (which is not healthy unlike a steady weight loss) and exercising more (which could also be dangerous), but BEWARE: your body sense that you are not eating much, and instinctively panic that there is a famine. It will promptly slow your metabolism right down so you store more of the food you do eat as reserves, so that you don't become too thin (and therefore ill or worse) during said 'famine'. You can't fight this natural process. Then if you start eating more when a goal weight is reached, your metabolism will be so slow that the weight will pile on. This is why people report regularly that they put weight on so quickly after a diet; they've done it too fast and now have to start all over again. Here we have the classic scenario for the' yoyo' dieter. Times when people may want to lose weight quickly could be before a wedding or big event, to prepare for baring all in a bikini on summer holidays, or perhaps they have signed up to take part in a marathon or sporting event and need to get trim and fit. Much better to plan ahead for these occasions and take it slower over a longer time. But if you must lose weight quickly, support your new eating habits with plenty of weight-bearing exercise, such as walking, dancing and weight training – this tones muscles, and the more muscle you have the faster your metabolism will be. Be careful when increasing your calorie intake to maintain your weight as your metabolism will be much slower and you may need less food than you think.

Weight versus inches

Muscle weighs more than fat. A person who is lean and toned will weigh more than a person of exactly the same size who has little muscle tone. If you are exercising whilst (or instead of) cutting calories you may be gaining muscle as you burn fat. This is a very healthy way of getting slim and fit, however it would be easy to get disheartened if the scales aren't saying you've lost much, and you may even gain a small amount weight at first as you tone up. If this is the case, you'd be better off measuring your achievements by measuring your waist, thighs, buttocks, upper arms or wherever else you want to lose weight from, taking note of how your clothes are getting looser. You will gradually go down clothes sizes and be toned and glowing with health too!

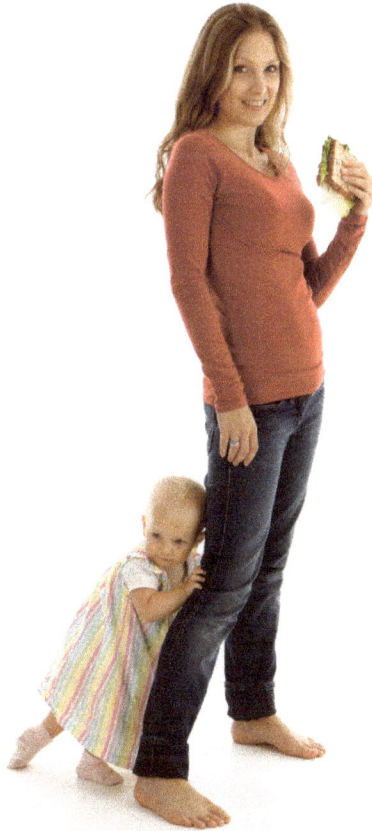

2 Motivation

Some people who want to lose weight find they cannot do it. There are various possible reasons for this. The first is medical conditions and medications that make them gain weight, in which case they must see a doctor or specialist about this. The second reason is lack of education, people genuinely not knowing how many calories foods contain or what it is that is making them put on weight. That is what I am addressing with this book – I hope to show people why they can't lose weight, and how simple and effortless it can be when you know how. The third reason is motivation, or lack of it. People know they shouldn't sit in front of a movie and devour an entire box of chocolates, yet they still do it. They know that a huge slice of chocolate fudge cake with chocolate sauce and ice cream for pudding is not going to do their waistline any favours, but that doesn't stop them having it. As with all addictions, I believe that you are not going to change unless you really want to. You have to have a reason for changing, whether that is something specific such as those listed below, or simply that you really feel that now is the time to change.

So let's say you have decided to make changes to the way you eat. Congratulations! However, I'm sorry to say that is probably not the end of it. There will be times when you can't be bothered, or when temptation gets the better of you. But that's OK, because nobody can be perfect 100 percent of the time. As this book will tell you, this way of 'normal eating' involves no deprivation and you shouldn't feel hungry, or feel you are missing out. Without even realising it you should gradually lose weight, your clothes will get looser and with it your body confidence will hopefully increase. Once you know how that feels it should be all the motivation you need.

Why do you want to lose weight?

The obvious answer is that you need to because you are overweight, but why now? If you have only recently gained weight and want to get back into your old clothes, then have a think about what you were doing before to stay slim, and what you are doing now that is different and making you fatter. This happens for many people over the Christmas period, and drastic dietary measures or intense fitness regimes really aren't necessary if you didn't have a weight problem before – just go back to your pre-Christmas healthier eating habits.

Recently having a baby is another reason you may be heavier than you have always been. You should always wait at least six weeks and get the all clear from your GP before losing weight after giving birth. If you have always been big, then there are bound to be more ingrained habits for you to break and changes to a way of eating that you might have had since childhood.

Trying to have a baby is a reason to lose excess weight. Having a BMI which is too high or low can result in little or no ovulation, without which conception is unlikely to happen naturally. The *British Medical Journal*[5] found that very obese women (BMI 38+) were less likely to conceive than women of a healthy weight, particularly women who carried their weight around the waist (apple-shaped). Being very overweight while pregnant is also linked to gestational diabetes and pre-eclampsia, two conditions which can be very dangerous for both mother and baby if not kept under control.

If you are getting married, be realistic about how much you can lose safely before the wedding, and the more time you give yourself the better. Crash diets will only leave you looking pallid and exhausted on your big day when you should be glowing and remember your fiancé fell in love with you for who you are, regardless of your weight.

Baring all in a bikini or shorts on a summer holiday makes many people cringe at the thought of their body being exposed, so you are far from alone here. The pre-summer holiday diet plans and products available are now as prevalent as post-Christmas ones, with companies cashing in on people's desire to lose a few pounds quickly. Losing weight for a holiday is as good an inspiration as any, providing you don't try and lose too much too fast, as crash diets can be dangerous and at the very least are unhealthy. Try to plan ahead to give yourself plenty of time to reach your target weight before you set off. Of course, if you return to your old eating habits when you get home as there is no longer a holiday to prepare for, you will only regain all the weight you have lost. See *Chapter 5, Where Are You Going Wrong?*, for more on eating while on holiday.

If, like me, you are already a parent, I'm sure you will empathise with the wish to do the best you can for your children. This involves setting standards for them to adhere to including with their food intake. I'm sure most parents would prefer their children to eat a healthy, balanced diet than sugary, processed snacks and drinks. The best thing you can do is to be a good role model. Children like to copy their parents, older siblings and or other role models they have in their life. I know my daughters would rather eat the same as me every time; if I'm eating an apple they'll want one, and likewise if I'm eating cake they'll also want some! They'll eat most things as I've never given them 'baby food' as such, just chosen sugar- and salt-free options and made sure they get all the nutrients they need (young children need a greater percentage of fat in their diet than adults and should get plenty of calcium as well as other vitamins and minerals). They're happy to try anything if we're eating the same thing. It's my job as a parent to set an example, not only what they eat but also how and when, and how to behave at the table. However, one thing I will not do is force them to eat if they're not hungry. They still have the instinct of knowing when they're hungry or full that so many adults have lost, and I don't want to mess with that. This is not an excuse for refusing what I've made for them because they doesn't like the look of it (this probably rings a bell with most parents of toddlers!); if they're genuinely hungry, I know they'll eat it, so I'll just wait another half hour or so and try again with the same plate of food. I'll put bets on them finishing the lot! It would be easy to throw the rejected food away and end up giving them unhealthy snacks later when they ask but that is an unhealthy pattern I do not want them to learn. And I won't give them snacks just before a meal for obvious reasons. If they're really complaining of hunger then at least I know they're going to finish all of the home cooked, healthy meal that I have made, and there will be yoghurt and fruit on offer if they're still hungry afterwards. Snacks in between meals are fruit, especially bananas for energy, or 'healthy' biscuits, breadsticks and cereal bars such as sugar and salt-free toddler ones or ones we've made at home together, but they also have to know that treats are allowed in moderation so occasionally we have an ice cream or piece of cake in the afternoon together, with a cup of tea for me and a glass of milk for them. I make sure they have fun playing outside in the garden on the slide and trampoline by playing with them or tidying the garden while they play, and they help (or try to!) clean the house, all of which keeps me active and is setting yet another good example. There is a place for TV, and quiet time for reading books is really valuable time together where they can learn a lot, but it is not good for adults or children to sit in front of the 'telly' all day. There are more games consoles, internet-based activities and home entertainment systems around than ever before, so it's no surprise that according to the Child Growth Foundation, children's waistlines have expanded an average 12.5 cm since the 1970s![6] In a nutshell, if you want your children to be fit and healthy then you have to show them how, by doing exactly that yourself.

Diagnosis from a doctor of a condition such as high blood pressure, diabetes, heart disease or another weight-related condition is sometimes the wake-up call people need to get their act together when it comes to their diet. (High cholesterol levels can also be found in people of a healthy weight and is thought to be partially hereditary[2], but diet and lifestyle changes can make a big improvement – if weight is not an issue the emphasis is on changing to different foods, notably less saturated and hydrogenated fats, rather than less calories.) If not managed properly these conditions are can be serious if not fatal, so delaying changes to your diet and lifestyle is just not an option. You should always get advice from a doctor if you have any medical condition before making dietary changes or taking up more exercise. Once you've been given the go-ahead, and if you have not been given a specific diet to stick to, then you cut calories in the same way as anyone else, using the tips in this book. However as your health is also at stake and your body is possibly in less than perfect working order there needs to be more emphasis on healthy, wholesome foods that will help heal your body, and less on saturated and hydrogenated fats, as well as cutting calories. See *Chapter 9, A Balanced Diet*, for more on healthy eating.

Perhaps you simply want to become, or get back to, a healthy weight, to get fit and to look and feel great. Well that's the best reason of all as it means that whatever else is going in your life, even with no holidays or weddings to plan for, you still have the same goal regardless. Joining up with a friend who also wants to lose weight to keep each other motivated can be a good source of support and encouragement at the start, but once you've reached your goal weight you have to maintain your new habits regardless of the other person, who for all you know may regain the weight or you may lose touch with them for whatever reason. Ultimately you have to do this for yourself and with every little step you are making progress even if the scales don't show it yet, so you should be proud of yourself. I can't imagine getting that same feeling of pride after weight loss surgery, as much as some people do believe it is the right thing for them. It can't possibly give you that proud feeling of 'I did this, all by myself'. You can do it, and you will be proud of yourself!

Why now? I never make New Year's resolutions. Not because I'll break them, but because if I want to do something I'll do it now. I appreciate that this is typical of my (Sagittarian) star sign, and that I am a self confessed impatient perfectionist, an all-or-nothing person, who wants everything done yesterday and done perfectly at that! If I haven't already started something or at least started planning or researching then I know my heart probably isn't in it. These aren't always good character traits – I can drive my family mad with my demands and have had to learn to be more patient – but it's this drive that, amongst other things, got me finishing this book! My point is that whilst not everyone is such a strong and driven character (and this is not a criticism, you are much easier to be around for long periods!), everyone has some strength in them, however deep it may be buried. Grab that strength by the horns and go for it. Don't resort to phrases such as 'Tomorrow never comes' or 'The diet starts on Monday'. You've heard them all before for a reason. START NOW! Or at least at the next meal – if you've already cooked it just eat less that you normally would and have some extra vegetables or salad to fill up. If you plan ahead and set a 'D-Day' date you'll only dread the day coming. You may get into a negative frame of mind and it will demotivate you. Plus you'll probably eat loads over the days before as your pre-diet 'last supper', so may even gain a bit more weight that you will have to lose. With the way of eating described in this book, there is no need for that last supper as you won't be giving anything up. So go for it!

Make a list of reasons you want to lose weight and keep it folded in your purse. That way you'll never be without a little inspiration.

Why did you stop 'dieting'?

Did you only plan on losing weight for an occasion such as a big party or wedding? What now? Did you return to your old way of eating, thinking (or hoping) that this time your body would react differently and not turn those extra calories into extra weight? Perhaps you intended to continue, but without the pressure of an upcoming event gradually slipped back into old ways. After all, years of habits might take more than a few weeks or months to break.

Perhaps you were doing well until an unforeseen event threw you off track – a family crisis, change of job or home, going away to university or moving in with a partner. It's understandable things are going to change in some ways, like how and where you shop for food, who does the cooking, how often and where you eat out. Maybe you don't have as much time as you before for planning ahead and cooking healthy meals, or eating healthily just hasn't been a priority.

If you were losing weight to look good on holiday, or went on holiday whilst in the middle of trying to lose weight, did you plan to allow yourself to eat whatever and whenever you liked on holiday? It's perfectly OK to relax a little and enjoy all the lovely food on offer whilst on holiday, but continue to eat like that when you get home and you are bound to gain weight. See *Chapter 5, Where Are You Going Wrong?*, for more on eating on holiday.

Often people 'fall off the wagon' purely because they become bored, depressed, stressed and demotivated. They get fed up of eating things they don't like whilst depriving themselves of food they love. They don't enjoy food the way they used to, can't find things they can eat at restaurants so stop going out, and their whole life seems to revolve around this new eating 'regime'. They can't wait to reach their goal weight so that they can eat what and when they like again, failing to see that this is how they became overweight in the first place. Most often the diet is stopped even before a goal weight is reached.

One friend told me that they 'stopped focusing 100 percent on the diet' (due to stress). This is due to an instinctive reaction from both your body and brain which kicks in to stop you from dying of starvation, a very real threat in the years of the paleolithic man when food was scarce and every day was spent hunting and foraging for food just to survive. You don't eat enough, so your body thinks (rightly) that you are starving, and assumes this is due to a natural famine, because of course humans can't possibly be stupid enough to deliberately starve themselves? So your primeval instincts kick in and your priority is finding food – you think about it, dream about it, plan what to eat, devise recipes, wander around food shops, study restaurant menus, constantly tempting then depriving yourself. This isn't crazy behaviour, this is your body's biologically instinctive way of trying to get you to eat.

This scientifically proven physiological reaction is why so many 'dieters' fall of the wagon; they get too hungry, and usually end up overeating the wrong foods to compensate (often high in sugar, fat and refined carbs to boost energy). Listen to your body (see *Chapter 16, Learn to Listen*)! If you are eating correctly your body will not be starving, you will feel satisfied and energised, and will naturally come to a healthy weight. Your body and brain will not be in 'starvation mode' so you won't need to think constantly about food. A blessing really – how difficult it is to not eat when all you can think about is food! Try also to find other things in life to focus on. Perhaps you can engross yourself in a project at work or take up a hobby for evenings. Maybe spend more time doing quality things with your family, even if that simply means fifteen minutes doing a puzzle or some colouring with the kids. Don't watch too many TV shows based around dieting and/or cooking and try to keep meals simple for a while so you don't spend all day cooking (unless you genuinely enjoy this!). It's hard to be surrounded by food and not end up picking at it constantly. These tips probably don't have to be followed for very long, just until you get more comfortable with eating normally and can be around food without feeling the need to eat everything you see. It may be helpful to plan ahead what you are going to cook or eat, and write it down so you can stop thinking about it and simply refer back to your list when you need to. Sometimes if I've had a busy day I forget to think about or don't get round to planning what we are having for supper until it's actually time to eat, but that's no excuse for eating unhealthily. Baked beans on wholemeal toast, omelettes and fresh soups are often on the menu in our house.

Identify your demons

When do you overeat? There are probably patterns in your weight and eating habits that coincide with what's going on in your life, and this applies to people who undereat as well as those who overeat. Identifying these patterns and devising alternative strategies is a great help in getting through times when you would normally turn to food.

Boredom can lead you to think about food and eating, and this in turn makes you hungry – we all know how a good TV advert for a yummy food product makes your tummy rumble! If boredom makes you eat then find something to distract yourself, it's amazing how quickly the (false) hunger passes. Have a drink in case you are mistaking thirst for hunger, and get stuck into something that you can make last until your next meal. Go for a walk, do the washing up, check your emails, phone a friend, whatever works for you!

Stress and depression is another common reason for overeating. The need for love and comfort is universal, and comfort eating starts the day we are born and are given our mother's breast or a warm bottle when we cry. Babies use milk as a source of comfort as well as for nutrition, and this behaviour continues into later life, when unfortunately we learn to turn to high fat and sugar foods (breast milk is naturally sweet and high in fat), so cakes, biscuits, chocolate and junk food give us an instant feeling of warmth and comfort. Unfortunately this is then followed by guilt, more depression, weight gain and more stress, so eating not only fails to solve the problem but also aggravates things by adding on more pounds to lose on top of everything else you may be dealing with. By dealing with the real issue at hand – trouble at work, relationship problems, family stresses etc, you can help solve the real reason you feel bad without turning to food. Keeping a journal of your feelings, calling or meeting up with a friend or family member to chat, or doing something you enjoy such as treating yourself to a massage are starting points. Getting some fresh air and sun (wearing sunscreen and following sun safety advice), taking some light exercise, and eating properly including foods with B vitamins are all proven mood lifters. The herbal remedy St John's Wort (read the label before taking) can help with mild depression, but if you think you need further help your GP can refer you to a counsellor and prescribe medication for severe depression.

Giving up an addiction such as smoking sometimes leads to a replacement activity such as eating. Smokers often report that smoking curbs their appetite, and having a cigarette in your break at work or with a coffee can be replaced by having a snack instead, so it is quite common for people to gain weight when giving up smoking if they choose food instead. Don't return to smoking, however – it causes mouth and lung cancer, as well as bad breath, poor skin, yellow nails... the list goes on. A heavy smoker is likely to be much more unhealthy (not to mention more socially unacceptable) than someone who is slightly overweight. If you are giving up smoking, place more importance on eating regularly low calorie, low GI foods to keep blood sugar levels steady, thus helping both hunger pangs and energy dips as well as nicotine cravings (see *Chapter 3, How Diets Work* for more information on low GI foods). Do something with your hands if you are used to holding a cigarette. Keep an elastic band on your wrist to play with and it's there whenever you need it. Try to stay away from other people while they are smoking, or you'll only make staying off cigarettes harder. And last of all add up all the money you would have spent on cigarettes and treat yourself to something which makes you feel good and reinforces the positive changes you are giving

Giving up smoking with another quitter never works since if one person falls of the wagon the other one follows. Integrate yourself with other non-smokers for company so you don't feel 'left out'.

your body – a facial, a new set of trainers so that you can do some exercise, or even just a really good book to curl up with for some relaxing 'me time'.

Poor body image is depressingly common, especially amongst women. Perhaps it goes back to our primal instincts to attract a mate. Our society's increasingly high standards don't help. We look to models and celebrities to inspire us, but these people have personal trainers and nutritionists, flexible working hours and childcare so that they can work out for three hours a day. However much a 'stick thin' celebrity claims they can 'eat whatever', don't believe them. They are normal people, not super-human, and they can only get that thin by eating only a little and exercising quite a lot. They can afford liposuction and other weight loss procedures, cosmetic surgery and other non-invasive procedures to keep them looking young. So we feel inferior for not being able to also achieve this.

Poor body image is obviously more prominent in people who are overweight and unhappy about it. I'll probably get a barrage of criticism for saying this but I don't believe those who are extremely overweight and say they are happy with it. Why would you be happy feeling tired and out of breath, not being able to buy or wear whatever clothes you want, and most importantly putting your life at risk? Fat 'role models' who embrace being very big (I'm talking obese here, not 'curvy' or a little chubby), stand up for bigger people's rights (such as free obesity-related healthcare etc), and even start their own plus-size clothing ranges, are quite frankly doing as much good as the (now banned) adverts promoting smoking. They are encouraging people by saying it's OK to be very overweight, to be (sometimes dangerously) unhealthy and putting their life at risk or at the very least risking all sorts of medical complications that would require lifelong medication and treatments.

Anyway, my point is that most people want to be slim and healthy. Yet ironically this low self-esteem is exactly what triggers a food binge! This causes more weight gain, poorer body image, lower motivation, a What's-The-Point and I-Don't-Deserve-It attitude, so more comfort eating.....and you see why people can get stuck in this cycle. Unrealistic, unattainable pictures of thin celebrities don't help; these people have money that funds personal trainers, chefs, dieticians, childcare, supplements, surgery...... there's no way most women can afford the time and money required to do what they do. Many of these so called role models aren't even healthy, and to be healthy does not require their extreme measures. However the more we are bombarded with these images of 'perfection' the worse our perception of ourselves becomes.

Unfortunately to break this cycle you probably can't wait to feel motivated, as that may never come. Making changes to the way you eat first, however, will prove to you that you can do it. Keep going and you will see changes in your weight and how you feel physically, thus proving you can do it. Feel your clothes getting looser, your energy levels getting better, and your enjoyment of life increasing. All this without depriving yourself of any foods and it should be much easier to maintain than previous fad diets you may have tried (and failed). You can do it! With increased energy and motivation for life you may even be achieving more; perhaps you are doing well at work or are getting more done in the house, catching up with friends you haven't seen or spending more time with your children. Look around at all the things you are achieving and increase the value you put on yourself as a person – you *are* worth it!

Deprivation, both physical and emotional, is a loaded gun for dieters. Filling an emotional void with comfort food literally 'fills the hole' left by loneliness, grief or loss. This loneliness, literally if you have few or no friends or relations, or psychological if you don't feel close enough to the people around you to share your feelings and problems, leaves people feeling bored and empty. Food becomes a friend, welcoming you home at the end of the day and keeping you company in times of need. Grief caused by loss of a loved one or even a close companion moving away is equally easily filled with food. Loss can come in many forms – the end of a relationship, falling out with a friend or family member, losing your job, even suddenly being stuck at home with a baby can make women feel like they have lost their own identity and sense of self, regardless of the fact that they love their baby more than anything. Food can temporarily fill these emotional gaps and provide comfort, not to mention purpose as preparing food and eating fills in time you would otherwise spend dwelling on how bad you feel.

As for food deprivation, I've discussed numerous times throughout this book how depriving yourself makes you crave food more. If you are hungry you will, of course, crave food. If you are missing certain nutrients you will crave them (or foods which temporarily satisfy these cravings). If you are depriving yourself of things you love then they become like the forbidden fruit and you will only want them more. Giving up carbohydrates completely will often result in a huge chip butty when you can stand it no longer. Resist a slice of cake for long enough and you might eat half a cake instead. I know you've heard it before, but it's true that a little bit of what you fancy does you good in more ways than one.

There's nothing to stop you taking your own drinks and snacks to the cinema. You'll be in control of what you're eating and will save a fortune!

Traditions and rituals such as chocolates in front of the TV, popcorn at the cinema, beer in front of the football or biscuits to dunk in your mug of tea may be so habitual you do them without even thinking, not stopping to consider if you are really hungry. If you are hungry and it's a while until your next meal, get something else to snack on which isn't so calorific. The obvious choice is fruit, but a cereal bar, small biscuit, or low fat yoghurt are healthy options. You can still join in with food elsewhere – a small amount of plain popcorn, just one or two chocolates from the box, a small scoop of ice cream or just one biscuit won't do much damage so long as you don't keep going for second and third helpings.

Social events can be hard to navigate for someone watching their weight. Wine is offered as soon as you step into someone's home for a drinks or dinner party, bars offer a far bigger list of alcoholic and sugary drinks than low calorie ones, and being taken to a smart restaurant and ordering lettuce is not exactly demonstrating you are enjoying the evening. So how do you cope when faced with less control over what's on offer? If offered drinks as soon as you walk in the door you don't have to be rude but gladly accept, then make the glass last as long as you can so hosts don't feel obliged to keep offering you more, and you don't wander around empty-handed. Go for low calorie choices whenever the chance is presented – there is usually water offered at any dinner party (the 'I'm driving' excuse works a treat), but otherwise just try not to drink too much (whilst drinking enough non-alcoholic fluids to stay hydrated, especially in hot weather).

Remember that unless you are socialising with friends every day then the odd occasion is not going to hurt. The same goes for food which your host has lovingly prepared – you don't have to finish every bite but you wouldn't want to be rude and leave too much, so just stay away from any optional extras such as bread and butter, cream on puddings and chocolates with your coffee. If you enjoy eating out at restaurants regularly then you can't get away with the most fattening option every time as you could if it was a rare occasion.

If you don't want to broadcast the fact that you're watching your weight then confide in one close friend who can back you up and support you when you're out.

There are always things you can order so watching your weight is no reason to stop going out, even in fast food restaurants (see *Chapter 15, Anywhere, Anytime*). In bars there are plenty of ways of joining in without consuming vast quantities of both calories and alcohol (see *Chapter 6, Liquid Energy*, for more information).

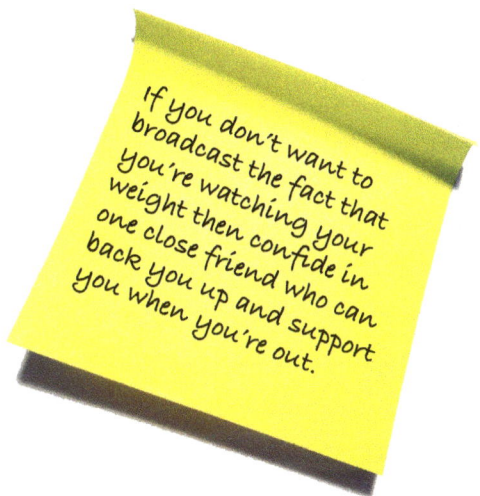

How can you get back on track after losing motivation?

You did it before, why can't you do it now? Well of course you can is the answer to that. Unless between then and now you have suddenly lost the power to think for yourself, buy, cook, and eat food with your own hands, then you have 100 percent control over what you do and are perfectly capable of choosing how, when and what to eat. Telling yourself you can't or have failed before is putting you in a negative mindset from the start, and making changes to your lifestyle seems like one long slog of deprivation and hard work. STOP! This is not a diet book, and you are not going 'on a diet' now. You are making small positive changes to the way you eat that will make you look and feel better both physically and mentally. You are doing this for life and will never need to look back and repeat the diet cycle again because you won't need to. By reading this book and following the advice you are not embarking on another 'regime', instead you are freeing yourself from the diet cycle so at last you can actually eat what you want to!

You are also a different person from last time, however recent that was. Slightly older, wiser, more experienced and more knowledgeable, you are better equipped this time, even more so once you've finished reading this book. As it is a lifelong way of eating there is no rush and you can make changes one day at a time, at your own pace, and are not being forced to overhaul dramatically everything you know overnight. You don't have to throw away what you have in the cupboards or ban certain foods from the house, you can still go out to eat socially and you don't have to spend any more money on food than you usually do or shop and eat at different places. You can do this because what I am advocating is realistic, flexible, normal eating, which absolutely anyone and everyone can do if they know how.

3 How Diets Work

Calories In = Calories Out

In other words if you eat more calories than you burn, you put on weight. If you eat less than you burn, you lose weight. Every diet works like this. Here are some examples:

Low carbohydrate

Meals consist of mostly or only protein such as meat, eggs, fish and sometimes pulses such as beans and lentils. Protein encourages the release of the hormone peptide YY which signals to you that you are full. If you eat meals based on protein you will feel full sooner, so you will eat less (and therefore less calories), and also feel satisfied for longer, so you are less likely to snack (so less calories). People on this type of diet report feeling less bloated than when they eat carbohydrates while at the same time feeling satisfied after a meal. The common, sudden drop in weight after starting the diet is because dieters find themselves urinating often as the body tries to rid itself of an overload of toxic amino acids from eating mostly protein, showing as 'weight loss' on the scales.

Meal replacement products

Usually two meals per day are replaced with a ready-made milkshake, soup or bar, with a calorie-restricted meal once a day, and sometimes low calorie snacks in between such as fruit or small cereal bars. The meal shakes and bars tend to be around the 200 calorie mark. Two of these, two 100 calorie snack bars, and one 600 calorie meal add up to 1,200 calories per day, which most people will lose weight on. Cereal brands use this concept by advising replacing two meals a day with a bowl of cereal. The portion sizes on the box also equate to around 200 calories a bowl.

The Zone

This diet advocates a ratio of 40:30:30 for carbohydrates, (lean) protein and (unsaturated) fats respectively. This is said to balance insulin (the hormone responsible for balancing blood sugar) and therefore keeps energy levels steady thus reducing hunger pangs. This is also said to be a good ratio of food groups for overall health, which is no surprise seeing as it similar to the recommendations given by the Food Standards Agency (see *Chapter 9, A Balanced Diet*). Weight loss ultimately comes from the fact that if you follow the diet strictly (with portions stated in the books) you will be eating only 1,000–1,300 calories per day.[7]

Low fat

Fat is higher in calories than other food groups – 9 calories per gram compared to 4 calories for lean protein and carbohydrate. Fat is dense in calories so it is easy to eat a lot of calories without eating a large portion. Eating low fat versions of the same quantity of food will equate to fewer calories, so long as they don't contain higher amounts of sugar, which processed foods often do to make up for the lack of taste in low fat products.

Low GI (glycaemic index)

Foods are given a number which tells you how fast it is absorbed into the blood stream; the lower the number, the slower it is absorbed, and therefore the steady release of energy keeps you sustained for longer, dispensing the need to snack on high sugar foods. Low GI foods also fill you up quicker so you eat less in the first place, as they tend to be higher in protein, and/or fibre than high GI foods. The sugars in low GI foods also tend to be the slower energy releasing fructose rather than 'sugar rush' inducing glucose.

Detox

These vary enormously but usually involve reducing your food intake to fruit and vegetables and their juices, sometimes with a small amount of plant foods such as lentils and quinoa. When followed strictly their calorie intake is usually very low, resulting in weight loss. The diuretic and laxative effect of all the fruit and vegetables can display apparent further weight loss but this is purely to due to water loss and empty bowels.

Weight Watchers

This is similar to calorie counting, except foods are given a number of points according to the calories and fat in them. For this reason, if you stick to your given propoints (the lowest allocated being 26 per day, more depending on how much weight you've got to lose) you will lose weight.[8]

Diet pills

These work by suppressing appetite, reducing the absorption of fat in the bowels, speeding up the metabolism, or a combination of all three. Trials show they can help (ultimately what you eat and how much you exercise are the definitive factors), however placebos have proved to be equally effective in some studies.

Grapefruit diet

Eat half a grapefruit or a glass of grapefruit juice before each meal. Grapefruit is said to contain enzymes which aid digestion and burn fat when combined with protein. For this reason most meals are only protein and non-starchy vegetables although some versions allow restricted carbohydrates. It is probably also likely that you are full of (very low calorie) grapefruit and so eat less of your meal. Another common factor of the different versions available is the low calorie allowance – 800 to 1,000 calories daily, and let's face it, most people are going to lose weight on this amount.[9]

High fibre

Fibre fills you up very quickly and is often found in low GI foods such as oats and in particular the bran part of cereals (which make you feel fuller longer), and in fruit and vegetables which don't contain many calories. Eating this way will help combat overeating and therefore cut the number of calories consumed.

Food combining

This uses the principal that proteins and carbohydrates need different enzymes to be digested; proteins need acidic enzymes and carbohydrates need alkaline ones. By eating both at the same time the two enzymes cancel each other out, rendering digestion less effective. Partially digested food is then left in the intestine to be absorbed and deposited as fat, as well as causing indigestion and other health problems. Food combining meals consist of either protein or carbohydrates, with a minimum four hours between each meal. You are also instructed to have a diet based mostly on fruit and vegetables with small portions of protein, carbohydrate and fat, and to eliminate processed foods completely.[10]

Raw food movement

As the name suggests this way of eating consists of only raw foods, or food not heated above 92°F–118°F depending on the food in question, in order to preserve nutrients and more specifically enzymes, which raw foodists champion for their various benefits to health and digestion. It excludes all cooked and processed foods and all food should be vegan and organic, so no animal products or derivatives. Foods which are inedible raw such as rice and grains can be 'sprouted' by soaking in water, and some recipes require food to be 'dehydrated' in a kitchen appliance devised for this, to form foods with similar tastes and textures to cooked food. Called a 'movement' rather than a 'diet' as it is a way of life for followers, weight loss is often cited as a common benefit. This is mostly due to the vast majority of the diet being low calorie, low GI, and high fibre, so it fills you up, keeps you feeling satisfied for longer, and keeps blood sugar steady.[11]

Fasting Diet

Involves eating normally (whatever you want within reason, bingeing on three tubs of ice cream in one sitting would probably not count as reasonable!) for five days a week, then restricting calories to 500 a day for woman or 600 for men. 'Fast' days can be any two days, and you can have your small calorie allowance in any way you wish, though foods high in fibre, water and protein are recommended as these are the most filling.

How Diets Fail

Let's get this straight; most diets don't 'fail' if you follow them correctly – you will lose weight. But wouldn't it be ideal if we could just eat well in the first place then not have to bother going on some radical 'diet'? Most diets are not realistic plans that you can effortlessly follow for life and some can actually be very unhealthy long term. Think about it, if everything the diet industry sells and promotes worked long term, they would all be out of business as no one would be overweight. Here are my reasons for not wanting to waste my time (and money) on fashionable diets:

Low carbohydrate

This is definitely not healthy long term, as are any diets that entail missing entire food groups, as you will not receive all the nutrients your body needs so will not only be malnourished but also may end up craving them more which isn't helpful when you are trying to avoid them. Short term problems reported include low mood, lethargy, headaches, constipation, and bad breath. Although studies are still being debated about the exact risks of a high protein, low carbohydrate diet, some professionals propose an increased risk of osteoporosis, kidney problems (from excess protein) and damage to other vital organs, atherosclerosis (fatty deposits in the arteries which can lead to heart disease). Anyway a life without toasted sandwiches and roast potatoes is not worth it in my opinion!

Meal replacement products

Most commercial processed shakes and bars offer little nutrition compared with fresh, balanced food of the same calories. They can also be expensive, and difficult to continue on holiday, with friends and at restaurants.

The Zone

The 40:30:30 proportions for carbohydrates, protein and fat for this diet are sustainable long term but calculating the meals to be in exact proportions is time consuming. Using it as a rough guide, the balance is not bad but the low calorie allowance is not realistic unless you are extremely inactive, very elderly or bedbound.

Low fat

Low fat does not mean low calorie, it is possible to overeat and put on weight with a virtually fat free diet. A diet too low in fat will be boring, unsatisfying and unhealthy.

Low GI

Low GI doesn't necessarily mean healthy. A jacket potato has a higher GI (85) than milk chocolate (49)[12], but a potato is more nutritious. Also while this diet will help curb your appetite it will not stop you from overeating.

Detox

Definitely not sustainable long term, both in terms of the restrictions on food groups and the low number of calories consumed. Even as a short term diet (some advise three days) the health benefits are still undecided by health professionals.

Weight Watchers

I'll admit it's hard to go wrong if you follow all the advice and stick to your tailored points allowance. However dwelling on the number of points in everything that passes your lips can become obsessive, so work out what are healthy portions from the guides, such as for the size of a potato, bowl of cereal etc, and eventually you will learn to do this automatically.

Diet pills

These could be dangerous if taken long-term. Their ability to increase weight loss is debatable when placebos have been shown to be equally effective, suggesting that the healthy diet and exercise advised with most pills are the actual reason for weight loss.

Grapefruit diet

This is probably not harmful short term but a bit tedious having to eat so much grapefruit and definitely not compatible with eating out at restaurants or friends' houses. It is still possible to overeat if you don't reduce the amount of calories consumed on top of the fruit. The restrictions on the types of food allowed could also mean missing out on certain nutrients.

High fibre

This diet usually gives calorie guidelines for losing weight, so simply by sticking to the recommended calorie intake you could lose pounds without following the foods advised. Without following these guidelines it is still possible to put on or not lose any weight as it is still possible to overeat high fibre foods. This is quite a healthy diet although excessive fibre consumption can cause diarrhoea and so interfere with nutrient absorption, and in most cases the gas and flatulence experienced are less than pleasant!

Food combining

Any diet that tells you to have a diet based mostly on fruit and vegetables with only small portions of protein, carbohydrate and fat is going to reduce calorie intake, however and whenever you eat them. A four hour gap between meals also reduces the opportunities for snacking. Evidence is inconclusive as to whether combining protein and carbohydrates has any effect, positive or negative, on your overall health or weight.

Raw food movement

Many typically high calorie foods such as processed and junk food, commercial cakes, burgers, sweets etc are banned from the diet, so this immediately reduces the opportunities to over consume calories. Most of the foods advocated are low in calorie (fruit, vegetables, salads, sprouts) and high in fibre (grains, beans and legumes, nuts and seeds), which allow you to eat bigger portions without the calories, and keep you feeling satisfied for longer. The highest source of calories comes from the oils in plant sources such as nuts and seeds, avocados, olives and vegetable oils. Because calorie counting is not required, it is possible to overeat raw foods and therefore gain weight.

Much of the fibre in fruit and vegetables is found in the skin, so wash the food thoroughly and eat without peeling first.

Fasting Diet

Do the maths. Eat 3,000 fewer calories a week (which you would be doing if you ate only 500 calories two days a week, based on a 2,000 calorie requirement for weight maintenance), and you are clearly going to lose weight, with or without any additional physiological changes which may or may not be going on. One thing we do know is that going without food releases large and often detrimental quantities of stress hormones such as cortisol which can themselves cause problems in other areas of health.

Add ingredients to reduced fat mayonnaise to make other dips, such as mixing it with tomato ketchup and lemon juice to make a seafood cocktail sauce.

4 A Quick Guide

Dos and Don'ts

There are some things that can be learnt from all the dietary information we are bombarded with, after all there are genuine reasons why you do lose weight while following them. Of course, they ultimately all come down to cutting down calorie intake, but the tactics they use can often be incorporated into a 'normal' way of eating to help you cut calories from your daily food.

Unfortunately there are also many nonsensical myths when it comes to losing weight so it's no wonder we, as a nation, have become confused as to what we should and shouldn't be doing. One minute fat is the evil ingredient, the next minute carbohydrates are banned, while I remember a phase when even vegetarians claimed it was their dietary choices which kept them svelte. Fast food chains have also been blamed and, can you believe it, actually sued for making people fat! What did they do, drag customers through the door and force food down their throats?

Here are some of the things you may have heard before, but note what headings they are under – some things are worth listening to and following, while others are either speculative myths and not worth bothering with as their benefits are so minimal, or just plain silly.

What can we learn from different diets?

So following these diets is not always advisable but let's take the elements that make the diets work and see if they can be incorporated into our daily life and a lifelong eating plan.

- **Protein suppresses your appetite**. Try to incorporate it into every meal.
- **Calorie restricted meals and snacks can help.** Look at the labels. Is there a lower calorie version you might like instead? For example, reduced fat mayonnaise.
- **Eat a balanced diet** with the right proportions (in the right amounts) of all the food groups will give your body all it needs. If your body has all it needs, it will not ask you for more food.
- **Fat is high in calories**. If you want to eat fatty foods without gaining weight you will have to eat less of them; one teaspoon of mayonnaise instead of one tablespoon, one or two sausages instead of three etc.
- **Foods with a low GI rating** will fill you up quicker and make you feel fuller for longer. Some also come with other benefits such as the vitamins you get from wholegrain varieties.
- **Fibre fills you up** and keeps you full for longer.

- **Low calorie, watery foods** such as fruit, vegetables and salad vegetables are bulky, filling and provide many vitamins.
- **Restricting calories** (and exercising to burn them off) is the only proven route to weight loss.

There is no need to count calories meticulously, or even at all, as the system does not suit everyone and if done rigorously it can become time consuming and obsessive as there is so much to remember. Losing weight should not interfere with the rest of your life. But you do need a rough knowledge of whether different foods and meals are high, medium or low calorie depending on their content and portion size, to be able to cut your calorie intake. This, along with exercise, is the only way to lose weight.

Tips to reduce calories

Upon reading these you will probably think you already know most of it as they are common sense really. On the other hand, if you can hand on heart say you always remember and follow them, you probably don't have a weight problem and so aren't reading this book! So here are some reminders to help you back on track:

- **Grate cheese** rather than slice it – you'll probably use less.
- **Trim visible fat** off meat before eating, and remember that meat and poultry skin is very high in (saturated) fat.
- **Fill up on vegetables**, and have small amounts of fattening foods along side. That way you feel full, don't miss out on foods you love, and don't consume too many calories.

Make a habit of filling half your plate with vegetables or salad before adding other foods.

- **Use 'reduced fat' or 'extra light' versions** now of the usually high calorie mayonnaise and vegetable spreads. Personally , I can't tell much difference between these and their full fat counterparts, but they are much lower in fat and calories in comparison. Though try to avoid ones full of additives and artificial ingredients. There is a huge array of fat free or low fat (and therefore lower calorie) salad dressings on offer too.
- **Read labels** and get to know which ingredients are low in calories. Vinegar (all types), lemon juice, herbs and spices, tomato ketchup, Worcestershire sauce, soy sauce, mustard, and mint sauce are some examples of foods which, when

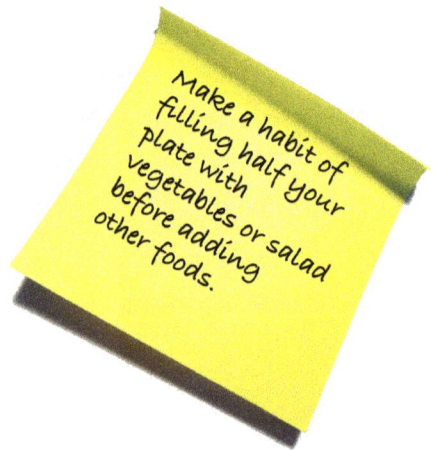

used in normal amounts, are low in calories. Highly flavoured foods such as garlic and chilli are another way to perk up dishes, as are strong flavoured ingredients that you only use a very small amount of such as Parmesan cheese and anchovies.

- **Profit from your own educated knowledge** for portion sizes – some packaged foods suggest portions that are large, making you buy more as they hold fewer servings per pack, but use nutritional labelling to guide you (also see *Chapter 14, The Diet Plate*). On the other hand some products advertise themselves as 'diet', however their low fat and calorie calculations could be for very small portions (commonly the case with cereals). Use your own common sense if you think a label is misleading

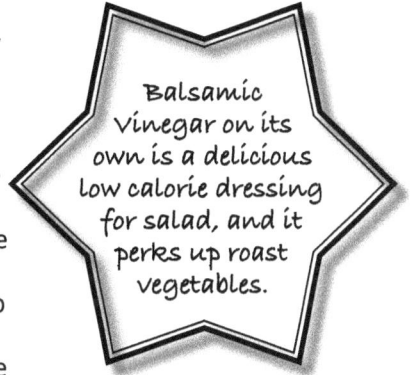

Balsamic Vinegar on its own is a delicious low calorie dressing for salad, and it perks up roast vegetables.

Tips to ignore

A week doesn't go by without another magazine or celebrity boasting about a new magic trick to lose weight, ranging from the obvious (eat from a smaller plate) to the downright ridiculous (eat something the size of a 50p piece every fifteen minutes) to the quite frankly scary – the Tapeworm Diet involves swallowing pills of the parasite which then eat away at the contents of your intestines! They are all completely unnecessary when all it takes is a normal healthy diet to stay in shape.

Here are some things I've read which I don't believe are worth the effort:

- **Drinking coffee speeds weight loss**. Caffeine in coffee, cola and energy drinks has been shown to increase metabolism (the rate at which your body burns energy). The effects are minimal and not worth bothering with (coffee is also diuretic in high intakes and can cause headaches and blood sugar swings).
- **Chilli and cayenne peppers** have also been shown to increase metabolism. Again, the effects are minimal.
- **Adding lemon juice or vinegar** to food decreases the glycaemic value (see GI diet in Chapter 3). Perhaps, but will your food taste nice? Again, a negligible difference.
- **Eat small portions**. Well that depends on what it is. Vegetables, fruit and salad are filling with minimal calories, so eating large portions of these will fill you up and prevent you from overeating high calorie foods.

- **Fibre eliminates calories**. It has been suggested that eating enough fibre flushes 245 calories out through the laxative properties. Not to be relied on, though fibre is good for overall health and will make you feel full quicker.
- **Being cold burns calories**. Your body does burn more to keep warm but only slightly, and being cold isn't nice! However you can accelerate the process of calorie burning by moving more, working harder and faster, whether it's walking down the road or hanging out the washing. You may feel more inclined to do this if you're not too warm as being active will increase your temperature. It has the added benefit of helping you get more done in less time too!
- **Smoking** has long been associated with weight loss for several reasons. Nicotine increases metabolism very slightly though not enough to make a noticeable difference. However, smokers do report less of an appetite so the amount they eat is less overall, without changing the type of foods they eat. Anyone who smokes or has friends who smoke knows that nicotine addiction is so strong that often cigarettes take priority over food, so if smokers only have enough money on them for a pack of cigarettes or a slice of cake, the fags will usually win.
Lastly, the coffee and biscuit combination that many of us enjoy is replaced by coffee and a cigarette, and since the national smoking ban came into place this means stepping outside the building and away from the office biscuit tin!
- **Eating at night makes you fat**. Not true, it's the overall calories you consume that matters, whatever time of day it is. What eating late might do is stop you sleeping or give you indigestion if you lie down. If you miss breakfast the next day to make up for it, you miss the metabolism kick-start that breakfast gives, and this may leave you tired and reaching for sugary junk food later.

Ridiculous tips to *really* ignore!

This is just a bit of fun to show how crazy and mixed up the world of dietary advice has become. When you consider food is really there purely to keep us alive, I wonder what our prehistoric ancestors living in caves would have thought of all this! Wherever you go people will talk about diets (mainly women though more and more men are getting in on the act too); what diet they are following; what diet their friend/Mum/ Pilates instructor is on; what diet celebrities swear by. It's something we all can share in common as, even without a weight problem, we all need to eat. It can be helpful to join up with a friend to talk, support each other and swap tips. However these absurd quotes were heard with my own ears coming from people I believe to be quite intelligent! It just goes to show that if you are desperate enough to lose weight you will believe and try anything, as these hilarious remarks prove:

I don't eat grapes because they are the most fattening fruit.

If you are overweight, I would hazard a guess that grapes are probably not the main culprit.

There are no calories in chicken.

The crazy remark from someone replying to the query of how many calories there are in a roast dinner.

It's the way the carbohydrates, proteins and amino acids work together in your body to make you burn fat which is why you lose weight.

Exclaimed by someone who was following a 'three bowls of cereal a day only' diet. Nothing to do with only eating 600 calories a day then.

Eating celery makes you lose weight.

So called 'negative calorie' foods are said to use more calories digesting them than they contain. Unfortunately this is not true, and anyway how much celery can you actually eat in a day?

Carrot cake is healthy as it contains vegetables.

So fruit and nut chocolate and apple pie must be 'good for you' too then? I'm not so sure either!

I need some advice, I'm really worried about putting on weight when I go to university as everyone always does.

I had to explain that you don't catch a 'university fat disease', and it is more likely the typical student diet of beer and too much junk food that is the problem!

C old food makes you burn more calories than hot food as your body has to use calories to heat it up.

Ice cream sundaes all round then.

T he calories in alcohol don't count as you burn them off through dancing and stumbling around everywhere.

They don't call it a beer belly for nothing.

D iet Coke makes you fatter than regular Cola because of all the artificial sweeteners.

Not true in the slightest.

I can eat what I like at the moment because I'm really stressed and stress burns calories.

If that were correct then Buddhist monks would all be very fat.

So, in conclusion, were any of these people successful in their attempts at losing weight?

What do you think?

5 Where Are You Going Wrong?

I feel frustrated when people tell me that whatever they do they can't lose weight when it really is so simple. But I realise not everyone has the same knowledge and experience to understand how calories can be accumulated without knowing it. When armed with this knowledge you are in control of what you consume, and ultimately being the weight you want to be is in your hands. In this chapter I've listed some common misconceptions about food that lead people to take in more calories than they intend to.

Pour sparkling water over a fruit tea bag and leave to brew for a few minutes for a refreshing drink with no artificial ingredients and virtually no calories.

Drinking calories

Newsflash – drinks have calories! I went to a well-known coffee shop recently with an overweight friend. I had a small cappuccino and she had a large mocha with whipped cream. Need I say more? It doesn't have to be this extreme. 'Healthy' smoothies and juices have more sugar and less fibre than whole fruits, and are surprisingly calorific. Regular cola has 140 calories per 330 ml can and orange juice has 149 calories for the same size can, though it does of course contain vitamins. The sugar in squash drinks has calories as does milk added to tea and coffee (though the amount of semi-skimmed milk required in two or three mugs a day won't be enough to gain weight – just watch the cream). The mistake of drinking calories seems to be such a big one that I have dedicated a whole chapter to it. Read *Chapter 6, Liquid Energy*, to find out more.

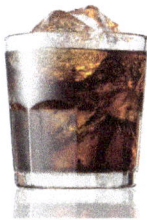

Cola
330ml / 140 calories

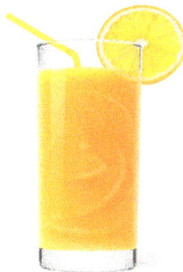

Orange Juice
330ml / 149 calories

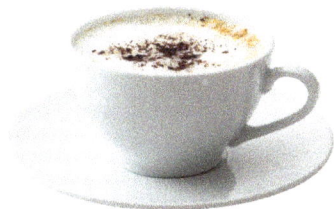

Cappuccino
80 calories

Hidden calories

Eggs scrambled with butter and cream look and taste much the same as when made with neither, but have far more fat and calories. Butter on vegetables and in mashed potato, oil in dressings and mayonnaise in sandwiches often go unnoticed but can contribute significantly to calorie intake. Similarly, some 'healthy' foods are still high in calories; avocados, olives, olive oil and nuts are full of goodness but are also high in fat so eaten in excess will contribute to weight gain.

Tuna Mayonnaise and Cucumber Sandwich 498 calories, 26g fat

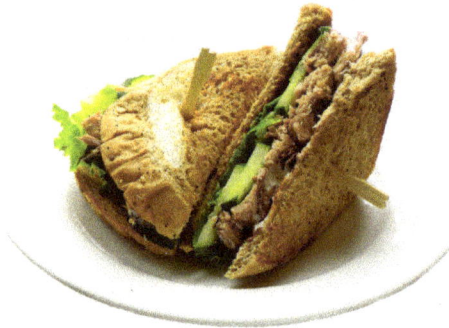

Tuna and Cucumber Sandwich 285 calories, 4.7g fat

Lack of 'movement'

I call it movement instead of exercise because as a busy Mum I don't have time for formal exercise, but I do the washing, cleaning, cooking, ironing, racing round the supermarket, not to mention playing ball in the garden and bouncy castle sessions at toddler playgroups! This year I've also finally got into gardening after at last buying my own house, and while I'm no botanist (and a self-confessed 'indoor girl') half an hour of weeding and raking in the fresh air and sun makes me feel fantastic. All of these activities use muscles and burn calories, and even get my heart rate up if I put enough effort into it (which has the added bonus of getting the job done quicker). If you like exercise then this won't be a problem for you, but I personally hate exercise just for the sake of it. I find it boring. I'd much rather do something fun that just happens to be exercise such as a dance class or a walk with my Mum and daughters.

Eating only low fat or 'diet' foods

As we've already seen, it's calories not fat that puts on weight. If you eat too much 'diet' food you will still put on weight. I once knew a colleague who was trying to lose weight. She would eat a jacket potato with tuna (no mayo or butter), low fat cereal bar, diet yoghurt and fruit every day for lunch. However the potato from the workplace canteen was huge, with a mound of tuna. Portion size plays a major part in the number of calories consumed as do too many extras – she would be better off dropping the cereal bar. For big appetites a side salad (watch the dressing) would do. Needless to say she never lost weight.

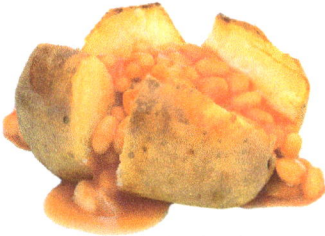

Despite being virtually fat free this 400g potato with 300g beans contains 459 calories

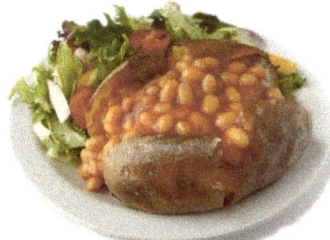

Whereas a 200g potato with 200g beans and an undressed side salad contains 326 calories

Low fat does not even mean low calorie because the calories may come from other sources such as sugar or carbohydrates. Boiled sweets are virtually fat free but their high sugar content makes them as calorific as chocolate. Remember it is calories that count. The same can be said of some cereals and cereal bars, and diet versions of biscuits and puddings. Below are some examples of 'diet' foods on the left, compared to 'regular' foods on the right, which in fact often have fewer calories than the diet products!

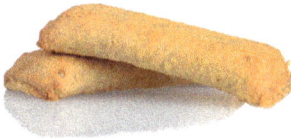

Baked cereal bar, 3.5g fat, 131 calories

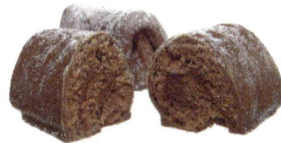

Chocolate mini roll, 5.2g fat, 113 calories

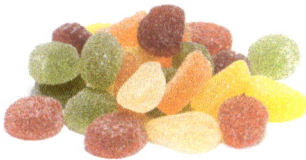

1 tube of chewy fruit pastilles, nil fat, 187 calories

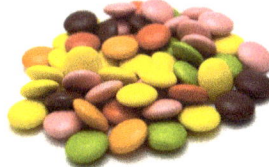

1 tube sugar coated chocolate buttons, 6.6g fat, 174 calories

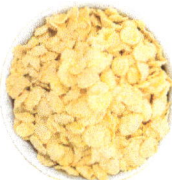

Low fat flakes, 40g bowl, 0.6g fat, 149 calories

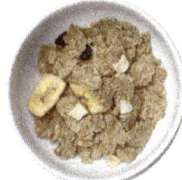

Fruit and Fibre cereal, 40g bowl, 2.5g fat, 143 calories

Unconscious eating

I hear so many people describe their daily food intake as fairly modest, and yet if they were to write down everything that passed their lips they would find a glass of juice downed as they ran out the house to leave for work, a 500 ml bottle of lemonade sipped throughout the morning, a biscuit from the staffroom tin, a chocolate from the box that was being passed round, leftovers from the kids' plates at teatime and two mouthfuls of a companion's pudding when out for supper. All forgotten! It is easy to see how the calories add up, and this is why keeping a food diary has been shown to help people lose weight.

Small portions (of high calorie food)

Have you ever heard an overweight person claim they didn't eat breakfast, only had a sandwich at lunch and soup for supper? They forgot the large caramel latte (364 calories) on the way to work and the large bottle of yoghurt-based smoothie (240 calories) they drank in the morning, and they didn't consider that the sandwich was a deep-filled chicken, bacon and salad at 610 calories. Then there was the can of cola (140 calories) and four chocolates from the tin brought to the office for Christmas (157 calories). The soup was half a carton of creamy chicken (283 calories) with which they had two slices of bread smothered in butter (400 calories), accompanied by a large glass of orange juice (150 calories). Total calories amounts to 2,345, but probably not very satisfying as the quantity of food isn't a lot. This isn't much more than the

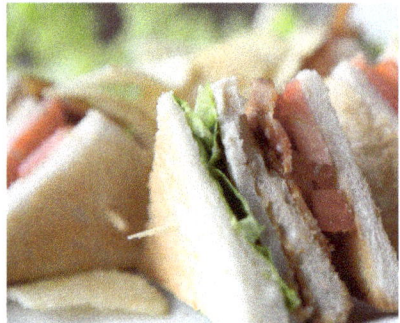

Chicken, Bacon and salad sandwich
29.9g fat and 610 calories

recommended daily allowance for a woman (2,000 calories) but with too sedentary a lifestyle this could add up to an extra ½ lb a week. It's not the physical size of the meal, but the calorific value that counts. In fact, large portions of lower calorie foods will fill you up and help prevent you from overeating more calorific foods. People are quick to point out how much I eat for my size, but if you looked closer it's often a lower calorie meal than it first appears.

Large portions

This should be common sense, but have you ever wondered whether you are just filling your plate up too much? Of course I mean with foods that contain significant calories; you probably won't be eating too much salad or vegetables and these wouldn't contribute to weight gain. I've often noticed female friends put on weight when they go from living alone or with parents to living with a partner. Upon witnessing food being served amongst these friends, it appears that everyone gets the same size serving. This wouldn't be so much of a problem if everyone was really in touch with their appetite and stopped when they were full, or were aware of their needs and the calories in food so chose not to eat all of it. However I very rarely see that happen, and it often means that a petite woman with a sit-down office job is coming home and eating the same portion size as a man. Lifestyle plays a part in a person's calorie needs; an office worker will burn off less calories than someone with a job where they are on their feet all day or someone doing manual work, or like myself running around after a young child! On average a man needs 2,500 calories a day whereas a woman needs only 2,000. The smaller you are the fewer calories you will need too, so short women (I mean fully grown, not teenagers who are still growing) need the least amount. It's no surprise that women put on weight if they are eating enough for a man! At home when cooking for my husband and myself, I have come to know very well how much we usually eat – with him eating roughly one third more than me depending on the meal (though sometimes if he's extra hungry he can eat twice as much!). Get creative with leftovers and you won't feel compelled to eat what's left straight away, or if you don't want to do this then cook slightly less and if it's all gone and you are still hungry you can always have some fruit or a healthy pudding afterwards.

It is also possible to reduce your appetite by not stretching your stomach so much every time you eat. The stomach is a muscle which stretches to fit around variable quantities of food then shrinks back to its normal size after the food has passed through (it is not possible to shrink the stomach to smaller than 'normal' without surgery). At some point during this stretching process your stomach and brain exchange messages to tell you that you are full. By eating less you may at first feel like you have more room, but over a few days your stomach and brain will adjust and you will feel satisfied with less quantities of food. Eating slowly will also give your stomach time to tell your brain you are 'full', making cutting the calories due to eating too large portions much easier.

I make crumble topping with wholemeal flour, oats, only a small amount of sugar and butter and sprinkle it very finely over unsweetened fruit. It's so healthy I sometimes eat it for breakfast!

Misleading names

Many products have misleading names, for example 'salad' does not mean low calorie. The word salad is defined as 'A cold dish of chopped vegetables, fruit, meat, fish, eggs, or other food, usually prepared with a dressing, such as mayonnaise'[13]. It only constitutes part of the 'fruit and vegetables' section of the Eatwell Plate (see *Chapter 9, A Balanced Diet*) if it consists of only fruit, vegetables and salad

Check portion sizes: If you were to look on the pack you might see that a bowl of low fat flakes may be advertised as having only 0.5g fat and 112 calories. Why? Because the serving suggestion is 30g whereas it is 40g for Fruit and Fibre.

vegetables. Salad ingredients such as pasta, potatoes, mayonnaise, dressing, croutons, chickpeas, kidney beans, couscous, coleslaw etc all add significant calories and should be counted as part of the overall meal, not dismissed as a calorie-free extra.

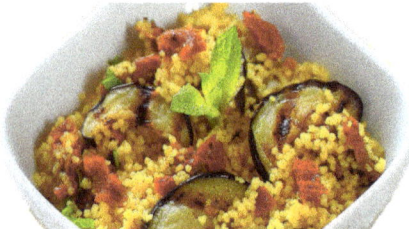

Chargrilled vegetables and couscous salad 200g, 8.6 fat, 253 calories

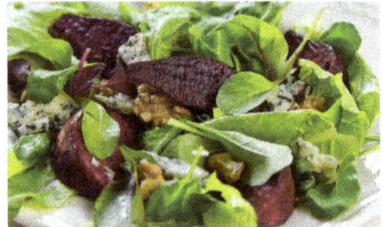

Spinach and beetroot salad 200g, 0.8g fat, 48 calories

Fruit crumbles, tarts, and 'wholesome' desserts such as rice pudding are often mistaken for being 'healthier' than their chocolate rivals but while there may be more vitamins due to the fruit content, at 600 calories for a restaurant serving of crumble it is far from waist friendly!

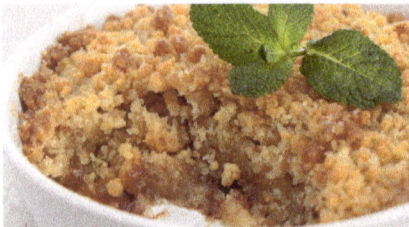

Apple crumble 600 calories

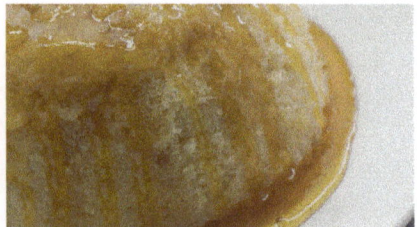

Treacle sponge 600 calories

Danger zones

I recently surveyed people about their real eating 'downfalls', situations where they know they definitely rack up the calories but have yet to find a solution feasible enough to follow. These are the answers that people came back with.

On holiday

Holidays are a chance to relax, as well as enjoy all the wonderful and exotic food on offer, not to mention having a break from doing all the cooking yourself! But this isn't the same as giving yourself licence to eat everything in sight, unless you are prepared to deal with the consequences of having to lose weight when you get home. You can still try everything, just don't eat too much of it. Have an ice cream, but make that your one afternoon treat, and save others such as cocktails, pastries and more ice cream for other days. Apply the same principles of portion control as you would at home, filling up on lower calorie vegetables, salad and fruit where possible, especially if there is a buffet where you have full control over what you put on your plate. Even out at restaurants the same applies as at home – the more calorie dense the food (oily curries, deep fried food etc), the less you eat.

Keeping active by walking round towns and markets, hiking in the countryside, water sports and digging sandcastles are fun ways of maintaining your activity levels while away from home. If you prefer to lie on the beach for two weeks that's fine too as relaxation is important, just be aware that you won't be burning so many calories so don't have too many high calorie drinks and snacks. Opt for low or preferably no-calorie drinks throughout the day, especially in hot climates as you will need to drink more than at home to keep hydrated.

Eating when drunk

A tough one, as whilst I could write the most brilliant advice here, chances are you won't remember it let along follow it at 2am when you're stumbling home. Aside from the issue of alcohol containing calories (if you are a regular drinker you should really take a look at *Chapter 6, Liquid Energy*), a person's logic, reason and sensible decision-making tend to go out of the window when drunk, leading to eating the nearest greasy, dirty, tasty food they can find. Food, especially fatty, stodgy food like the fast food people often reach for, helps line the stomach and recover sugar levels so it is actually a good idea to eat something after a night out. If you still have a vague ability to debate food choices as you step into the kebab house / chippy / burger bar then take a look at *Chapter 15, Anywhere, Anytime*, for suggestions on lower calorie choices at these food outlets. Alternatively prevention and preparation is the key. If you don't want to take a snack such as a cereal bar in your bag or pocket for your way home (and let's face it even if there was room alongside your phone/lipstick/purse in a tiny clutch, it would quite possibly get eaten, squashed or lost before you even set off home) before you go out lay out in plain view something healthy that takes little or no preparation, so that hopefully you turn to that when you return home. A healthy sandwich, toast, yoghurt and cereal are good options, or a couple of plain biscuits and a glass of milk. Don't forget to put out a jug of water and a glass – hangovers are in part dehydration and partly a build-up of toxins, so drinking plenty of water before you go to bed (two to four glasses should do it) will rehydrate you and flush out toxins, and help stave off feeling like death the next day.

Comfort eating

The need to comfort eat goes right back to when we were offered a warm breast or bottle of milk when we cried as a baby. Whilst this is needed for babies, as adults when we are looking for comfort it is not always food we need, though food is what we are craving at the time, and most often it is stodgy, fatty, sweet foods which replicate the rich milk we drank as infants. Usually arising from boredom, loneliness, stress and depression, food is often used as a substitute for stimulation, companionship and fulfilment. The obvious answer is to get to the root of the problem and tackle it, be it getting a new hobby or finding something else to do like tidying the garden or writing an email, phoning a friend or going to visit a family member, or taking some time to look after your emotional well-being by writing a diary of your feelings to clear your head or spending sometime pampering yourself to relax. For more serious depression it is essential you seek medical advice. In the meantime, instead of half a tub of ice cream in front of the tv, try a cup of tea with a biscuit to dunk, or a low fat instant hot chocolate drink. The warmth of a hot drink can be extremely comforting in itself, and you might find that was all you needed after all.

Tiredness

Not getting enough sleep encourages you to eat more. It makes sense, as the less energy you have, the more you will feel the need to eat during the day to get more energy. Unfortunately unless you are more active you won't burn off these extra calories, and it actually goes deeper than this. Professors at Stanford University, USA found that people who slept for five hours or less per night had 15 percent more of the appetite stimulating hormone ghrelin and 15 percent less of the hormone leptin (which lets you know you are full) than people who slept for eight hours[4]. Everyone has the odd late night but you can't go on with not enough sleep forever, so this needs to be addressed. Go to bed earlier even if the house isn't completely clean and tidy. Sleep before midnight is more healing and restorative than the same number of hours of sleep after midnight, so going to bed earlier and getting up earlier will make you feel more energised and healthy than if you stay up late[4]. This also follows our body's natural instincts to sleep when it is dark.

For the times when you are completely exhausted and a daytime nap is not possible, start the day with a good breakfast to kick start your metabolism which in turn will create more energy from what you have eaten and will burn reserve fat stores. Eat regularly throughout the day; three meals with a snack both mid-morning and mid-afternoon, and choose long lasting energy sources such as wholegrains, nuts and seeds, as well as protein to curb hunger. Avoid sugar which is not only calorific but will also result in an energy 'crash' after the initial rush, and do not overfill your stomach as trying to digest large quantities of food will only tire you out more.

Do not rely on caffeine as excessive consumption is not only addictive but puts your heart under stress as it makes it work faster. Caffeine stimulates the release of adrenaline, putting you in 'fight or flight' mode, making you feel alert. Essentially it puts your body under a state of stress, which is not a good thing. When it wears off you are left feeling more drained, tired and lacking energy, and the dip in blood sugar may leave you craving sweet (calorific) foods. In addition to caffeine, cola and energy drinks can also contain sugar and a cocktail of chemicals and artificial ingredients. However one or two cups of good quality coffee or two to four cups of tea (around 100–200 mg caffeine in total) per day are fine for most people. Avoid caffeine if you experience unwanted side effects such as anxiety, heartburn, headaches or an overly sensitive bladder, and some medications can interact with caffeine, so read the labels carefully. Don't drink caffeinated drinks in the evening or you may have trouble sleeping, so you'll be just as exhausted the following day.

Grazing

We are constantly surrounded by readily available food to nibble on: communal biscuit tins at work; packets of crisps and nuts in the cupboard; free tasting samples at the supermarket; the kid's leftovers; tasting food as you cook. It all adds up, and can amount to a substantial amount of calories over a day if you're not careful. You are more likely to graze if you are hungry, which is why it can be a good idea to split your meals into three main meals (breakfast, lunch and supper) plus a snack mid-morning, mid-afternoon, and before bed, avoiding hunger pangs by not going too long between eating, and keeping blood sugar levels steady. Blood sugar levels can also be kept steady by choosing foods which fill you up and give you long lasting energy such as wholegrains, nuts and seeds and fruit, rather than refined sugars which give you a 'high' followed quickly by a 'low'. Sit down for all meals and snacks, and keep 'nibbles' like crisps and nuts on high shelves so they are not so easy to get to. Say no thanks when the tin of chocolates is passed round for a third time, and take a healthy snack like fruit to have in your break at work instead of biscuits. Try not to cook so much if there are always leftovers, or turn them into the next day's lunch, saving money as well as your waistline! It's helpful to taste food as you cook it so you know the flavours are right, but that means a 'taste' not four mouthfuls! Also if you are not genuinely interested in trying or buying a product on display at the supermarket then you don't really need to eat the samples, which are often cold and dry by the time you get to them anyway!

Peer pressure

It's not easy trying to watch what you eat when all around you are guzzling like a pack of starving wolves. That's another reason I don't like strict diets, and a reason to continue eating normal foods, just in different amounts. If friends notice you are not joining in they may try to sabotage your efforts by telling you that one day won't hurt, or try and tease you into giving in. They probably don't mean any harm, and just don't realise how far you've come, and want 'the old you' back, the carefree one to bond with over a pizza and box of doughnuts on a Friday night. Firstly, they are right in that one evening of eating a little too much won't hurt if you are careful most of the time. But secondly and more importantly, why aren't you joining in? When you've finished reading this book you will see that you can eat pizza and doughnuts, and not low fat versions; you can eat the real, stodgy, fatty McCoy from your favourite takeaway. Just don't eat too much of it. There may be, however, people who become jealous of your weight loss, and your ability to stick with your efforts (they probably haven't read this book so don't realise how easy it is!). They may also try to get you to give in to make you less 'perfect', so they feel less inferior. Pity them, and offer them advice if they want it, but take jealousy as a compliment; you're obviously doing really well!

6 Liquid Energy

One of the most common mistakes people make when it comes to the calories and the energy they consume is not realising how many calories they drink. Wide-girthed men may refer to their 'beer bellies', but it's not only beer that makes you put on weight. Any drink that is made from anything except water, carbon dioxide, or sugar free sweeteners and flavourings will have calories, and therefore will contribute to weight gain if the person's overall calorie intake, including drinks, is more than they need. It is also easier to drink unconsciously, as you can have a bottle to swig from while you walk, a cup on your desk, and a glass in your hand at a social gathering without a second thought, whereas people are more likely to sit down to eat. For this reason people are likely to consume more calories than they intend to through drinks.

The act of chewing food signals to the body that you are eating and consuming calories, so your brain is on standby until you have consumed enough, when 'full' signals will be sent to your brain from your stomach, and you feel satisfied. As you don't need to chew drinks it takes much longer for this 'full' signal to be sent, by which time you have probably drunk more calories than you need and are drinking purely to satisfy thirst. If you are just thirsty, not hungry or needing an energy boost, choose low calorie drinks such as those listed below.

Different drinks and their calories

Milk

Milk contains calories, and while it also contains many valuable nutrients and is a very healthy drink as part of a balanced diet, you have to consider its energy value if you are watching your calorie intake. A chocolate milkshake at around 150–250 calories for a homemade milkshake made with powder and semi-skimmed milk, compared to 100 calories for 200 ml of plain semi-skimmed milk, can add pounds.

Do consider whether you really want to add those extra teaspoons of powder! Even adding virtually calorie free flavours such as coffee to make a latte does not discount the fact that the milk itself contains calories. There are now more milky drinks available than ever in our coffee shops, from cappuccinos and lattes to mochas, flat whites and hot chocolates, not to mention the flavoured syrups and whipped cream one can add,

Skimmed milk, whilst having fewer calories, does not allow you to absorb all the vitamins as you need some fat for this, so semi skimmed is better in nutritional terms.

and of course iced versions of all of the above. The increased variety on offer means that customers are no longer simply ordering a standard Americano coffee made with just espresso coffee and hot water (and a dash of milk, like the coffee you most likely drink at home). Whilst this is not necessarily a problem when drunk in moderation, these milky drinks do add to your daily calorie consumption, so take this into account when trying to lose weight.

Coffee

Just in case you decided to skip the paragraph above as you 'don't drink milk', but really enjoy a coffee, just what coffee are you drinking and how often? An espresso is a popular morning pick-me-up, or perhaps throughout the day for people who work long hours and need to concentrate! A coffee after a meal at a restaurant or dinner party is a traditional custom. Whereas coffee itself (and the water it is made with in an espresso or larger Americano) has only around five calories, turning that coffee into a milky latte, cappuccino, mocha, or iced milky variety adds calories surprisingly quickly when you consider that one small cappuccino is around 100 calories, with lattes and mochas being even more. Using sweetener instead of sugar does not make a lot of difference – a dash of milk and two teaspoons of sugar added to an Americano will still only be around 50 calories, and only around twenty if you don't take sugar. However sugary-flavoured syrups can add 60 calories to a small drink. Think before you order!

> If you really enjoy a milky latte, try using half water and half milk as a compromise – known in some coffee shops as a cafe au lait.

Ice cream shake

It should come as no surprise that milkshakes made from ice cream are high in fat and calories. However freshly made 'healthy' fruit smoothies can also be made with ice cream, making them misleading. Even low fat frozen yogurt alternatives can be pretty calorific. The best way to cut calories in milkshakes is to blend a smaller amount of the original drink really well with ice in a food processor and drink immediately before the ice melts. This gives the drink that 'slushy' ice cream texture without so many calories.

Fruit juice

Pure fruit juice is, obviously, the juice which has been either squeezed directly from fruit (advertised as 'not from concentrate'), or squeezed, dehydrated, then rehydrated by adding water (called 'from concentrate'). It takes more than one portion of fruit to make one glass of juice, so you get more (natural but still high calorie) sugar in a glass than in one piece of fruit. You also miss out on other nutrients such as the fibre found in the skin and pulp of whole fruits; however juices can be a source of vitamin C for those who don't eat enough whole fruit and vegetables. Fruit smoothies are puréed fruit, sometimes with added ingredients such as water, fruit juice, yoghurt or ice cream. They contain more health benefits because the flesh and pulp of the fruit is used as well as the juice, providing added nutrients and much more fibre. They still contain calories though, and it still takes more fruit to make a glass of smoothie than you would usually eat as whole fruit, so you are getting more calories and (natural) sugar than if you were to eat say, a just whole apple or peach, especially if extra juice, yoghurt, ice cream or sugar has been added. Smoothies are more filling than juice because of the fibre and thicker consistency and they can be a good breakfast or snack if the ingredients and calories are balanced and to your needs. It's when people drink them as a replacement for drinks like water that they can add extra calories.

Try half juice and half still or sparkling water as a compromise – the latter also is a good replacement for sugary fizzy drinks.

Yoghurt drinks

Yoghurt drinks are cast similarly to smoothies as health drinks (sometimes they are the same thing when both puréed fruit and yoghurt are put together). Yoghurt can indeed be very healthy – it can be very low fat, with lots of calcium, protein, and in live (natural) yoghurt there are friendly bacteria which support intestinal functions. However some are very high in (mostly saturated) fat, with lots of sugar and flavourings with very little real fruit and all contain calories in varying amounts, with fat content also varying between each brand. Like a smoothie, yoghurt drinks should be classed as a meal or snack on their own and not drunk just to quench thirst, which they actually won't do very well anyway as they don't contain as much water as other drinks. A new trend in the health food market is mini bottles of yoghurt drinks containing a 'daily dose' of friendly bacteria. These are lower calorie than larger bottles purely because of their size, and most tend to be low fat or fat free because they are aimed at a health conscious market. However, they still often contain sugar and do contain some calories, so just be mindful of this if you are restricting your calorie intake and don't swig them all day long!

Sugary drinks

The majority of the calories in fruit squash and fizzy drinks come from sugar. Squash is made from little or no real fruit juice. Some contain small amounts of fruit juice extracts, but all contain other flavourings (either natural or artificial or both) and sugar as well as possibly artificial sweeteners. It is the sugar which gives squash most of its calories. Fizzy drinks are made the same way but with calorie free carbon dioxide added, though they tend to have much more sugar than squash. Sports drinks are processed differently so you absorb more liquid (helping with hydration during exercise) than with other fruit, squash or water-based drinks, but most still contain lots of sugar. Diet drinks use low calorie sweeteners in place of sugar which, whilst better for the waistline, have been under intense scrutiny for the health risks associated with them. It is always better to try and wean yourself off having a sweet tooth, and don't encourage it in children.

If you must drink squashes always look for 'diet' or no added sugar versions, however due to the artificial sweeteners in them try to keep them as treats.

Alcohol

Alcohol contains seven calories per gram, almost as much as fat! This means that the stronger the alcohol percentage, the more calorific the drink will be. On the flip side, it is sugar which is turned into the alcohol, so the more alcoholic the drink the less sugar it should contain, as the sugar has been used up to make alcohol! However other calories can come from various sources depending on the choice of drink. Sugar is still present in most drinks but there is more sugar found naturally in beer than in plain spirits (without mixers). Alcopops contain fizzy sugary drinks not dissimilar to mixing a spirit with coke or lemonade. Liqueurs are basically spirits with added sugar, sweeteners and flavours, and creamy drinks (such as Irish Cream) contain sugar and cream (or similar milk-based products). Adding a fruit juice or non-diet fizzy drink to an alcoholic drink adds calories. Cocktails depend entirely on the individual ingredients; fruit juice, fizzy drinks, sugary fruit syrups, ice cream, cream, milk and chocolate sauce are just some of the ingredients which add calories to a cocktail.

On top of the calorie content, alcohol increases your appetite, and you are less likely to make sensible (and healthy) food choices once you have had a drink. Then alcohol actually slows the rate at which your body burns fat as burning alcohol is easier so takes priority.

However now to contradict myself! It is in fact better to drink alcoholic drinks with mixers instead of neat because when it comes to your health (and safety) calories are the lesser evil compared to alcohol. Drinking spirits with mixers, fruit juice or fizzy drinks, beer with lemonade (shandy) or wine with soda or fizzy water (a spritzer) means you are less likely to drink so much alcohol overall, will drink more slowly, and the water in the mixers will help prevent you from becoming too dehydrated (yes, alcohol is also a diuretic, another killer function). There are two ways in which you can cut your calorie intake while drinking alcohol. Either mix it with calorie free or diet mixers (such as diet fizzy drinks) without increasing the total number of drinks consumed, or, to comply with my advice throughout this book, just drink less.[14]

Non alcoholic drinks

Drink (average serving)	Calories per serving
Apple juice (200 ml)	100
Semi-skimmed milk (200 ml)	98
Lemonade (330 ml can)	132
Orange squash (250 ml when diluted)	70
Strawberry and banana smoothie (250 ml)	143
Mocha coffee (no cream, 8 oz or 250 ml coffee shop mug)	130
Low fat raspberry and yoghurt drink (250 ml)	193
Vanilla milkshake made with ice cream (12 oz or 350 ml)	400
Strawberry milkshake, semi skimmed milk, syrup, blended ice (12 oz or 350 ml)	235
Sports drink (500 ml bottle)	150

Alcoholic drinks

Drink (serving size and %)	Calories per serving	Alcohol per serving (units)
White wine (175 ml glass, 12%)	130	2.1
Beer (1 pint, 5%)	240	2.8
Whisky (25 ml, 40%)	55	2.4
Cider (1 pint, 5%)	200	2.8
Creamy liqueur (50 ml, 17%)	165	0.85
Non-creamy liqueur (50 ml, 40%)	160	2
Pina Colada cocktail	500	3
Alcopop (275 ml bottle, 5%)	154	1.4
Rum (25 ml, 40%) and Cola (150 ml)	126	1
Champagne (small 125 ml glass, 12%)	95	1.5

N.B. calories and alcohol units are approximations and will vary between brands.[14, 15]

Low calorie drinks

Drink (average serving)	Calories per serving
Water, still or sparkling (any quantity)	0
No added sugar squash (250 ml when diluted)	4
Diet cola (330 ml can)	1
Diet fizzy fruit drink (500 ml bottle)	16
Fruit or herbal tea, made with water only, (250 ml)	3
Coffee, instant or fresh, with 40 ml semi-skimmed milk	25
Black tea with 20 ml semi skimmed milk and 2 tsp sugar	42
Diet energy drink (250 ml can)	8
Low fat instant hot chocolate (11 g + 200 ml water)	40
Diet Tonic Water (150 ml)	3

As with food choices, you can of course drink whatever you like providing you don't exceed your daily calorie needs. Just bear in mind that liquids empty from your stomach faster than food so leave you hungry afterwards, even if you have just 'drunk' plenty of calories, and they don't offer as much nutritional benefit as most fresh food of the same calories. Just try to restrict calorific drinks to one or two a day; you probably won't miss them, and the rest of the time choose low calorie drinks. You won't feel any less satisfied, so cutting down on liquid calories is probably the easiest way to cut down on calories, and anything that is very easy certainly gets my vote!

7 Where Do I Go From Here?

If you want to reduce your calorie intake you have three options.

Option 1 – swap for different foods, such as:

Bag ready salted crisps, 11.7g fat, 183 calories **FOR** Banana 0.3g fat, 100 calories

Small mocha with whipped cream 10g fat, 200 calories **FOR** Small latte 4g fat, 110 calories

Pie, mashed potato, vegetables and gravy 36g fat, 900 calories **FOR** Quiche, salad 32g fat, 500 calories

Option 2 – change to a lower fat and/or low calorie version of a particular food, such as:

Chocolate mousse, 55g, 4.6g fat, 105 calories **FOR** Low fat chocolate mousse, 55g, 1.9g fat, 60 calories

330ml blackcurrant squash 143 calories **FOR** 330ml no added sugar blackcurrant squash 13 calories

150g Greek yoghurt 15.75g fat, 210 calories **FOR** 150g fat free Greek yoghurt nil fat, 78 calories

24g Cheddar cheese 100 calories 34.9g fat, 416 calories per 100g **FOR** 32g reduced fat Cheddar, 100 calories 21.8g fat, 311 calories per 100g

Cheddar photo 26

Fat is dense in calories so a low fat portion of a food will be bigger than a high fat portion of the same calories, which is useful if you have a big appetite. This means you can get away with eating the same amount of food while still cutting calories. Alternatively, you can eat more of that food without increasing the calories, as is the case with the cheese example above; useful for bigger appetites so long as you still don't consume too many calories overall.

Option 3 – eat smaller portions of the same food you always eat, such as:

A snack-size chocolate bar or half a larger one instead of a king-size bar. Or eat these foods less often – one large chocolate bar once a week has fewer calories than a small one every day.

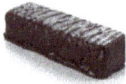

King-size chocolate wafer, 13.4g fat, 261 calories

FOR

Half or snack size chocolate wafer, 5.4g fat, 107 calories

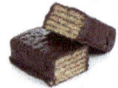

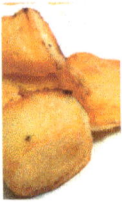

4 roast potatoes, 320g, 14.4g fat, 480 calories

FOR

2 roast potatoes, 160g, 7.2g fat, 240 calories

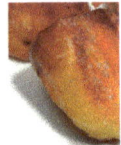

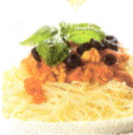

Adult restaurant portion pasta in tomato sauce with garlic bread 9g fat, 750 calories

FOR

Child restaurant portion pasta in tomato sauce with garlic bread 5g fat, 380 calories

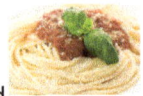

If you find it difficult stopping at only half a regular bar, buy snack-size ones.

Where *not* to cut corners

Cut too many corners and you risk missing out on vital nutrients. Some 'diet' foods are so full of artificial ingredients they can hardly even be called food and some just taste plain nasty. There has to be a limit on what and how much you cut out of your diet in your pursuit of cutting calories, or else your overall health and enjoyment of food will be compromised. Read on for some advice to make sure you don't cross that line.

1. We do need some fat, just the right amount of the right types (see *Chapter 9, A Balanced Diet*). Fat actually makes you feel satisfied quicker (and makes food taste nice) so you may end up eating much less of a higher fat meal than you would of a fat free meal.

2. Certain foods are not naturally low fat, such as mayonnaise. To recreate the same taste and texture in diet versions manufacturers often have to use lots of processing with additives. This results in a low calorie but somewhat artificial product with fewer nutrients. Some don't taste as nice as their full fat equivalents. This may be fine for you but you may prefer to just have smaller portions of regular products.

3. Some low fat products, such as cereal bars, are still high in sugar, so are no lower in calories than a bar with fat but less sugar. These fats are often in the form of nuts and seeds providing healthy fats, protein and fibre, so will ultimately be more satisfying, but without adding calories (see *Chapter 5, Where Are You Going Wrong*). The size of the bar makes a significant difference too, with some bars being 'diet' simply because they are very small. If you prefer the taste of bars that happen to be bigger you can always cut it in half.

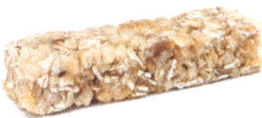

Low fat cereal bar 30g,
1.1g fat, 16.9g sugar 142 calories

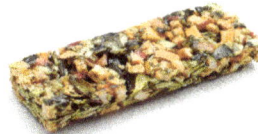

Nut and seed bar 30g,
3.7g fat, 9.6g sugar, 117 calories

4. Some vitamins, called fat soluble vitamins, actually need fat to be absorbed, so it is by no coincidence that these vitamins A, D, E and K are found naturally in foods containing fat such as milk, cheese, oily fish and avocados (vitamin K is found most abundantly in leafy green vegetables). As skimmed milk is very low in fat, the vitamins it contains are not as easily

absorbed by the body as they are fat soluble vitamins. Semi-skimmed milk has sufficient fat for vitamins to be absorbed, but full-fat has more fat than most people need so unless you genuinely prefer the taste of skimmed, go for semi.

5.   Quality can vary. Trying food alternatives is the only way you will find what works for you, but there are certain things I prefer. Reduced fat and half fat cheeses are a good swap as you probably won't notice any difference. However I have tried 'diet' and low fat Cheddar-style cheeses and personally don't like them; they are OK cold but they don't seem to melt or cook like full fat hard cheeses. Whether you go for them depends on personal preferences – I'd prefer to just use a smaller amount of full or half fat cheese.

Supermarket makeover

Three simple changes are explained at the beginning of the chapter, and all three will help cut your calorie intake and lead to weight loss. Which you choose depends on your preferences and circumstances – you may choose to eat all the foods you usually enjoy but just eat less of them, which does also save time if you already know where to find all of your favourite things in the supermarket.

On the other hand maybe you fancy a change and would like to try different things – maybe an obscure tropical fruit or a meal you've not cooked or eaten in a while. Finding low fat alternatives should be as simple as looking further along the same shelf – the low fat yoghurts are not very far from the full fat ones!

You could even make a note on your shopping list:

1.   Could I buy something different, with lower calories, instead?

2.   Is there a lower calorie alternative on this shelf?

3.   Can I make this packet last longer by eating less each time?

It really is so simple and easy to follow, and while you may have to think about what you are buying and eating at first, soon it will become such a habit that losing weight will happen without any thought or effort at all! Brilliant!

Old Shopping List	New Shopping List
Crisps	Dried apple 'crisps'
Whole milk	Semi-skimmed milk
Donuts	Bananas
Greek style yoghurts	Low fat yoghurts
Streaky bacon	Lean back bacon
Large white bread rolls	Small wholemeal rolls
Chicken Kiev	Marinated skinless chicken breasts
Multipack standard chocolate bars	Multipack treat-size chocolate bars
Large battered fish portions	Breaded fish fingers

8 Exercise

There are some people who really do relish exercise and enjoy working up a sweat as they pound the streets, feeling their lungs and muscles working and feeling they are fit and making progress. But I hate exercise. Or I think I hate exercise, or I at least hate the word 'exercise'. For me, it conjures up unflattering pictures of people, straining away in the confines of an over-air conditioned yet somehow still clammy aired gym. When I see people taking an hour out of every day to power walk round the same block of buildings six times before returning home, or paying through the nose to gain entry to what some might call a Torture Chamber (aka the gym), I think of all the things I would rather be doing – playing with my daughter, spending time with my husband, meeting a friend for coffee or even making a dent in the list of household chores would be preferable. And the money I'd save could go towards a family holiday or a nice romantic meal out with my husband (something that doesn't happen often these days!).

Now I'm going completely to contradict myself and say that I absolutely love dancing, whether it is learning a routine in a class or dancing with friends in a club or at a party (not that I have much time for either these days). I went to stage school and spent many years learning ballet, tap, modern, jazz, and street dancing like it was my sole purpose in life. Fast forward ten years and I no longer have the time or inclination to dedicate my life to dancing. Now I am a mother my life revolves around my daughters, who like most young children love a walk (or in their case a push in the buggy) around the harbour to feed the ducks. That's 45 minutes walking for me, and a blast of glow-giving fresh air for all of us. We live too close to the local convenience store to warrant using the car, so that's another twenty minute walk there and back every time we run out of milk. I join in at baby gym classes on the bouncy castle and kicking balls back and forward or pushing kids around in their sit-in plastic cars, and my daughters and I have dance sessions together in the sitting room with a favourite lively CD or dance DVD. After buying our first house I am determined to get it looking lovely, so an afternoon tidying the garden on a sunny afternoon whilst my kids play on the slide is fairly typical in the summer, and then there's the cleaning, sweeping, dusting, vacuuming and all the other energy expending chores, which are surprisingly satisfying once you can see the results. So I prefer to think of it as 'movement', all adding up throughout the day and contributing to my overall health and well being. Activities that just so happen to be physically energetic can be much more fun, and as long as you're not training to be a professional athlete they can provide all the exercise you need. There's no point in going hell for leather at something you loath purely to lose a little weight; all that will happen is that you resent it, stop doing it, reverse any benefits you may have gained and possibly be put off doing any kind of exercise in the future. If you are enjoying yourself you are more likely to continue. If you enjoy time to yourself in a gym or being pushed by a personal trainer that's great and you will benefit hugely. But if you hate it then that's fine too, there are endless ways you can get more 'movement' into your life that will help you on your way to being slim and fit.

So perhaps I do like exercise after all, just not in the conventional sense. I love the way fresh air and physical work actually make me more energised, and help me sleep better at night. The feel-good endorphins released during exercise are not a myth; they do actually exist, in the form of stress relief, increased vitality, mental relaxation and an overall feeling of increased positivity and happiness. If you've felt this before you'll know what I'm talking about. If you haven't then trust me it's worth trying to achieve.

Exercise doesn't have to be a part of losing weight as that can be done through cutting down on calories alone, but the calories burned during exercise will speed up your progress, and any increase in muscle mass will increase your metabolic rate. What is important to health is that you maintain a reasonable fitness level; strong muscles and bones, a healthy heart and lungs, and an all round well functioning body. Health professionals advise 30 minutes of exercise a day, five days a week but short bursts of exercise can be just as beneficial so long as you are getting enough in total.

As always, if you have any kind of medical condition, are pregnant, or are very overweight then you should get permission and advice from your doctor before taking up exercise, especially if you are planning on doing very strenuous exercise or have not done any exercise at all in recent weeks. Comfortable, supportive shoes appropriate for the activities you are doing should be worn, along with comfortable clothing. Being uncomfortable or too hot or cold will only put you off further exercise, which would be a shame as you may really enjoy it.

How much exercise do I need?

The Department of Health recommends 30 minutes a day, five days a week, of exercise that gets you slightly out of breath, raising your heart rate and body temperature.[16] This doesn't have to be achieved in precisely this manner; fifteen minutes twice a day (so long as you still get your heart rate up) or one hour a day for two days and half an hour on day three (providing that you are not too tired towards the end of the hour therefore making you perform

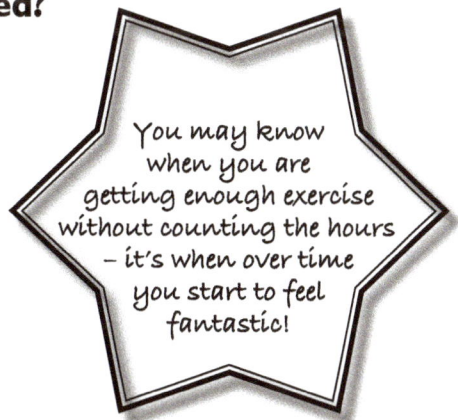

You may know when you are getting enough exercise without counting the hours – it's when over time you start to feel fantastic!

less efficiently) all add up to the same amount and should give you the same benefits. Many people achieve this without even realising – walking briskly to the bus stop or shops, climbing stairs and vacuuming all count towards this goal if you are putting in enough effort to get out of breath. Another recommendation is that you take at least 10,000 steps each day as an alternative way of accumulating enough exercise, as this is roughly equivalent to doing 30 minutes five times a week. Proven benefits of walking include reduced risks of diabetes, heart disease, dementia, and stress as well as improved heart and lung function and weight loss.[17] It is estimated that most people achieve 3,000–4,000 each day anyway just through their daily routine.[18] An easy way to monitor the number of steps you take is to buy a pedometer, which clips onto your belt or clothing so that it is in close contact with your hip, and counts the number of steps by the number of times you move your hip to take a step. Pedometers are available from many chemists and sports retailers as well as department stores, and start from as little as £1 for the cheapest to in excess of £100 for ones with other features such as heart rate and body temperature monitors, weather forecasts and remote connection to your home computer. They are relatively small and discrete and can be worn under most clothing throughout the day. You can increase the number of steps you take by choosing the stairs instead of an escalator or lift, parking further from your destination, walking to the local shops if you don't need to buy too much, going for a walk or going window shopping in your lunch break, and even changing the TV channel by walking to the television instead of using the remote! It all adds up, and if you don't do enough steps one day you can make up for it by doing more over the next few days.

You may have come across statistics stating how many calories are burned during a set number of minutes of specific exercises. I don't know where these statistics come from or who discovered them, but what I do know is that the number of calories burned per hour for different activities is as individual as how many calories a person needs to be a healthy weight. It depends on many factors such as age, height, weight, body fat percentage, muscle mass and general fitness. Then there are the circumstances which make even one person's results vary – the weather or how hot or cold you are is feeling, when and what you last ate and drank, if you have been ill, how tired you are, and of course how much effort you are putting into the activity. How much you weigh, your body fat percentage and how much muscle mass you have also affect metabolism (the rate at which calories are burned), and your values for these may be different from last week! But some exercises are generally better for burning calories than others. Running burns more than walking for the same amount of time (although walking the same distance, over a longer period of time will burn roughly the same, as the calculation is based on calories burned per mile or kilometre rather than time). Hiking on different terrains burns more, as does carrying a heavy rucksack (though take care not to hurt your back!). Cardiovascular exercises such as swimming, step aerobics, street or hip-hop dancing, cycling and football burn more per hour than gentler activities like yoga, golf, slow ballroom dancing, stretching and archery. It is common sense that the harder you have to work and the more out of breath you are getting, the more calories are being burned and the more your heart and lungs are improving. Other exercises can be just as beneficial for reasons other than burning calories such as muscle and bone strengthening, or improving balance and flexibility. See the list below for more on the benefits of different exercises.

Whether you choose a specific exercise routine, count your steps or just become generally more active in your day-to-day life doesn't really matter, so long as you are 'moving' enough you will be making a positive impact to your health and fitness and should not only see the results on the scales or how your clothes fit, but you should feel much better too, which I think is just as, if not more important.

Types of exercise

Aerobic exercise

Aerobic exercise is also known as cardiovascular exercise. It improves lung and heart function and promotes blood circulation which carries nutrients to where they are needed, aiding healing and building new cells to form skin, muscle and other tissues. Cardiovascular exercise enhances the intake, distribution, and use of oxygen around the body. This type of exercise is also good for fat and calorie burning so is ideal for people wanting to lose weight. Cardiovascular exercises should get you slightly out of breath, increase your body temperature which can make you sweat, and get your heart rate up. Brisk walking, running, swimming, dancing, cycling and climbing stairs are all examples. Impact training such as jumping, running and skipping are also great for increasing bone density.

Strength and resistance exercises

These tone and build muscle, improve the capability of muscles and the bones beneath them. Aches and pains such as a bad back are often due to weak muscles. Strengthening muscles also increases the body's ability to burn fat as muscles contain more mitochondria (the 'fat burning' part of a cell), so people with more muscle have faster metabolisms. Keeping your muscles strong as you age is a good way to help prevent developing a 'middle age spread', as muscle loss as you get older is the primary reason for a slowing metabolism. Also good bone density will help prevent diseases such as osteoporosis which can lead to frequently and easily broken bones. Resistance training requires you to only 'resist' a force, such as resistance bands (essentially a very large elastic band), light weights, resistance training machines found in gyms and fitness centres, and your own body weight while doing press-ups or sit-ups. Body-building uses similar exercises but the goal is muscle definition, shape and possibly bulking-up muscles. This is achieved in part by using heavier weights for fewer reps (repetitions, or number of times you 'lift' a weight), whilst strengthening exercises essentially use lighter weights or source of resistance with more reps.

Flexibility exercises and activities

These include stretching to improve the range of motion of the joints and muscles, resulting in a better range of movement. Sometimes these exercises are prescribed after recovering from an injury that has resulted in lack of movement for some time such as a fracture, which has caused the muscles around the injury area to stiffen. Improving flexibility also helps to improve posture, deep breathing, and relieve stress. Yoga, Pilates and gymnastics can also help, but simply stretching each muscle group in turn and holding for a few seconds every day is the simplest and easiest way to improve flexibility.

Good balance

This should be a by-product of strong muscles and bones, but these can get out of sync due to muscle wastage caused by age, a sedentary lifestyle or injury. Other factors such as poor vision, low blood pressure, vertigo and inner ear infections can also cause balance problems. Muscle strengthening exercises will therefore help improve balance and yoga, Pilates, walking, and ballet are all good ways of doing this. Walking also improves co-ordination, as does bouncing on a trampoline (mini-fitness ones as well as full-size trampolines), and dancing helps with co-ordination and memory. There are also numerous simple exercises you can do to improve your balance, such as standing on one leg and walking in a straight line placing one foot in front of the other, which can be done anytime and anywhere.

Make it fun!

Make sure you are comfortable – being too hot or cold or having sore feet are not going to make you want to continue!

There is absolutely no point in forcing yourself to do something which you hate. You will be miserable, resent it, give up, and possibly be put off taking up other forms of exercise in the future. As with changes to your diet, be realistic and honest about what you want to achieve and how you want to do this so that you don't end up 'failing' or falling short of your expectations. Better to take it slow then increase your levels of activity as and when you are ready rather than jump into the deep end only to realise you are out of your depth and pushing yourself too hard to reach unrealistic expectations.

Exercise doesn't have to mean a slog on the treadmill or braving the cold in winter. Perhaps you've always fancied trying out a form of dance or trying something new and exciting like surfing. As David Walters said, 'An hour of basketball feels like fifteen minutes. Fifteen minutes on the treadmill feels like a weekend in school traffic.'[19] You don't have to commit long term – changes to what exercise you do will give you different benefits, so if you try surfing and horse riding only for the one week you are on holiday then you can still go back to your usual activities upon returning home, with hopefully another skill under your belt for future holidays! Any sort of walking is exercise; shopping, looking round a museum or zoo, even walking to your local pub (providing you don't drink your weight in alcohol and calories when you get there!).

Maybe you've got a friend who would also like to go to a class with you or come for a walk – knowing you'll be letting someone else down can be an incentive for turning up, though you need to be doing this for yourself and want to go anyway in case it's them who lets you down. As an extra incentive you could finish with a (low calorie) drink or snack in a café as a nice way to the end your workout, and have a good chat at the same time.

Even housework can be made more appealing – turn on some upbeat music and go a bit faster as you do your household chores – you'll get the work done in less time and it won't seem like such a bore. Have fun washing the car with the kids or do those DIY jobs you've been meaning to get round to, you'd be surprised how much energy you can burn with a hammer and screwdriver.

Get going!

Getting started on anything new, especially one which requires physical as well as mental effort, can be daunting, and without an element of fun, escapism and achievement the word 'exercise' makes many people want to curl up back in bed.

It sometimes helps to have a goal to work towards such as a charity marathon you have signed up for or a competition or event meeting for whatever interests you. There are usually options for all levels of competence and you get to meet people with the same interests.

Joining a local club is also a good, non-competitive way of meeting people with the same

Eat shortly after exercising, and allow at least an hour after eating before exercising.. Exercising on a full stomach could give you indigestion, but eating after will replenish energy stores and help repair muscles.

interests. You can play with or against each other (depending on your choice of activity) or go for walks and make dates to do certain classes or activities together, compare techniques and pick up tips.

Most local leisure centres and gyms will have a huge variety of classes on offer, some of which are drop-in though others you may have to book ahead if they are busy. Once you know what you enjoy you can sign up to a weekly session for a term or longer and really improve your skills. Again here you will meet more like-minded people with similar interests and goals and may really begin to look forward to your weekly class as precious 'me time'.

If you think you can stay motivated without other people involved then how about setting your own goals? Maybe you increase the number of steps or miles you walk or run each day to reach a certain number by a set date. Or perhaps you pledge to try one new activity each week – you don't have to continue with it if you don't like it but at least you've tried. If you have more specific health concerns then perhaps your aim is to reduce your blood pressure or cholesterol levels by a certain amount, and of course ultimately lose the extra weight that is probably the reason for reading this book! Write your goals down and put them somewhere you can see daily, for example, on the fridge. Plotting your progress on graph paper so that you can track improvements is a great way to acknowledge even small changes, and seeing these will keep you motivated to carry on.

However you 'get going' with exercise, the most important factor is to not give up, which is why it is so important, like with dietary changes, to take up only what you know you can fit into your life. Far better to do only a little bit of activity for life than to do three hours a day for a week then sit on the sofa for the next month. That is not to say your goals and expectations will not fluctuate as your life changes. We all have times when we are more or less busy and in these times you have to be flexible and adapt. But if you tweak your activity habits to fit around your life, then you can continue getting the benefits of exercise and movement without compromising on everything else. Life shouldn't revolve around keeping fit; rather, you keep fit so that you can enjoy life.

9 A Balanced Diet

The eatwell plate

Use the eatwell plate to help you get the balance right. It shows how much of what you eat should come from each food group.

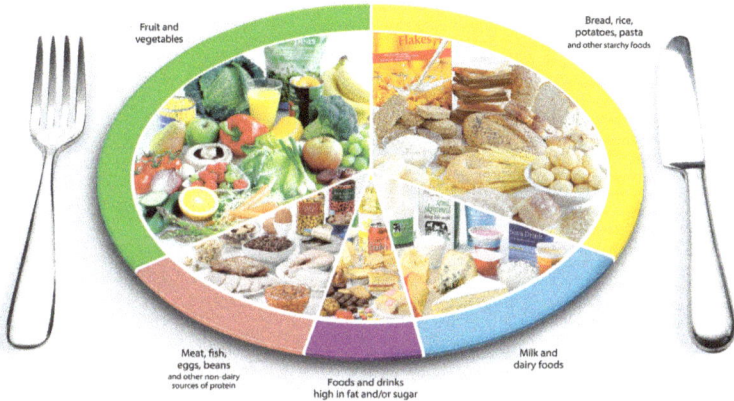

Fruit and vegetables

Bread, rice, potatoes, pasta and other starchy foods

Meat, fish, eggs, beans and other non-dairy sources of protein

Foods and drinks high in fat and/or sugar

Milk and dairy foods

Public Health England in association with the Welsh Government, the Scottish Government and the Food Standards Agency in Northern Ireland

© Crown copyright Public Health England in association with the Welsh Government, the Scottish Government and the Food Standards Agency in Northern Ireland.[20]

Carbohydrates

These are needed for energy. A minimum 47 percent of our diet should be from this food group (between 6–11 portions a day); of this 40 percent needs to be complex carbohydrates and no more than 10 percent simple sugars. Complex carbohydrates include pasta, potatoes, rice, bread, oats, cereals etc. Vegetables are also a source of carbohydrates, though not as good a supply as starchy carbohydrates. Wholegrain varieties also provide fibre which keeps your bowels healthy, lowers cholesterol, and regulates blood sugar. Wholegrains also have more nutrients and fibre than refined white grains and have lower GI, and potatoes with their skins on are better than skins off for the same reason. Sugar is a form of carbohydrate, including the natural sugars in fruit (see later section on *Sugar*).

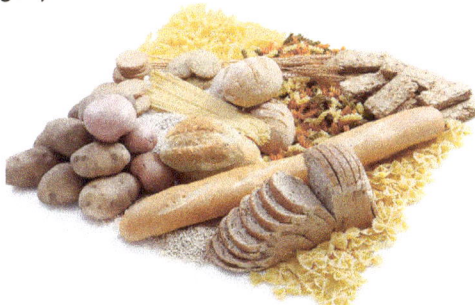

A portion of carbohydrate is:

- 3 tbsp cereal / 1 Weetabix or Shredded Wheat / 2 tbsp muesli
- 1 slice bread or ½ bread roll or ½ pitta bread
- 1 small pitta bread or chapatti
- 3 crackers
- 2 egg sized potatoes / 1 ice-cream scoop of mashed potato
- 2 tbsp uncooked rice or pasta (4 tbsp cooked)

Protein

Protein sources include meat, fish and eggs and there are vegetarian alternatives (see below). The Department of Health recommends eating 2–3 portions a day, including at least two of fish a week, one of which should be oily fish such as sardines, mackerel and salmon. Processed meat products such as burgers, sausages and fish cakes also count but can be higher in fat than lean, unprocessed meat, and are often mixed with other foods such as wheat, potato or breadcrumbs so are not always the best source of protein. Dairy products such as milk and cheese also contain some protein, but dairy products are counted as a separate food group.

Vegetarian alternatives include: tofu; micoprotein (such as Quorn); Textured Vegetable Protein (TVP); beans such as kidney beans; pulses such as lentils; nuts and seeds. However these are not as rich in zinc and vitamin B12 as animal protein so are not classed as 'complete protein'. You can create 'complete protein' meals by combining the above foods with grains such as wholegrain bread, pasta, and rice. Rice with black beans or peanut butter on toast are two 'complete protein' vegetarian meals.

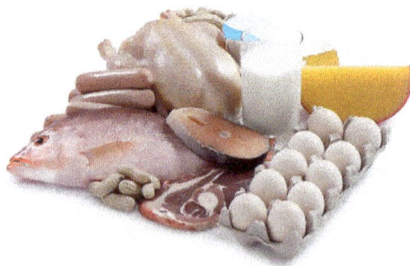

A portion of protein is:

- 50–70 g cooked beef, chicken, pork, ham, lamb, liver, kidney; oily fish, Quorn or tofu
- 100–150 g white fish
- 2 eggs (up to 6 each week)
- 3 tbsp baked beans, cooked pulses or lentils

N.B. Girls and women of childbearing age and women who are pregnant or breastfeeding should have a maximum of two portions per week of oily fish (a portion is around 140 g). Boys and other adults should eat no more than four portions per week.

Children, pregnant women and those trying for a baby should avoid shark, swordfish and marlin because of high levels of mercury in these fish (other adults should eat no more than one portion per week).

Fat

Fat Fact – we *need* fat. Far from being evil the right sorts of fats (in the right amounts) are necessary for health, and our diet should contain 20–35 percent total fat.

Unsaturated fats are the best and good sources of monounsaturated fats are nuts, avocados, olives and olive oil. Omega-3 polyunsaturated fats are found in oily fish, nuts and seeds. Omega-6 polyunsaturated fats are found in sunflower oil and other oils commonly used in food manufacturing. For this reason we need to try to eat more omega-3s and less omega-6s.

Saturated fats in meat and animal products (also cakes, cheese, biscuits etc.) should be limited to no more than 11 percent of your diet.

Hydrogenated fat (hardened vegetable fat) and trans fats (the result of partially hydrogenating vegetable fats) are the worst culprits and are found in margarine, pastry, biscuits, chocolate and similar processed foods. These should be limited to 1 percent of your diet. Many manufacturers are eliminating hydrogenated and trans fats from their products so if in doubt check the labels. You should be able to find similar yummy treats which are free of trans fats.[21]

A portion of fat is:
- 1 rounded tsp butter, margarine or spread
- 2 tsp low fat spread
- 1 tsp cooking oil e.g. vegetable, nut or seed oils
- 1 tsp mayonnaise or oil based salad dressing
- 1 tbsp cream

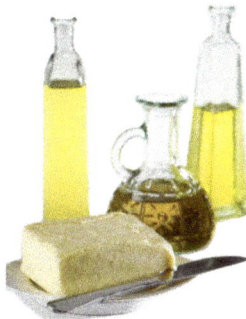

Sugar

Many brands of biscuits, cereal bars, yoghurts and snacks intended for babies and toddlers are sweetened with fruit juice instead of sugar and contain only wholesome, natural ingredients. They taste good too!

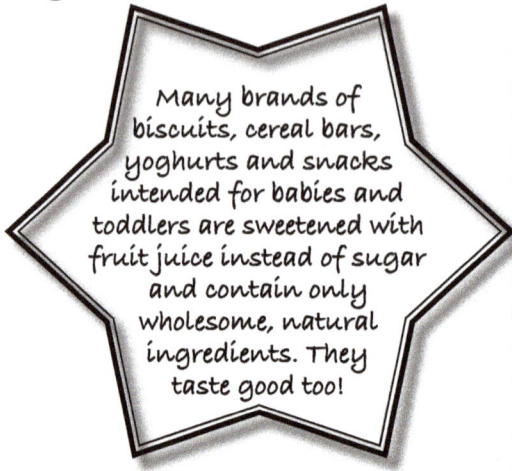

Sugar is a type of carbohydrate and in the form of sweets, jam, honey, chocolate etc. should be restricted. This is because they can cause rapid highs (and lows) of blood sugar (hence the energy rush they give) and insulin, that may contribute to the risk of diabetes and other illnesses. Sugar is also high in calories and contributes to tooth decay. High sugar content usually equates with a high GI rating, and simple sugars tend not to be very filling (with the exception of being eaten in fruit), making them not very helpful to dieters.

A portion of sugar is:

- 1 scoop ice cream
- 1 small (snack size) chocolate bar
- 1 rounded tsp sugar (for drinks), jam or honey

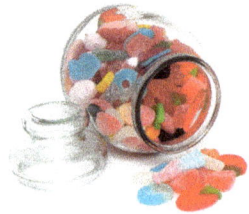

Fruit and vegetables

These supply vital vitamins (including vitamins A, the B group, C, E and K), minerals and fibre, and they can help towards keeping you hydrated as they often have a high water content. They also contain some carbohydrates. Five portions (a portion is roughly 80 g or what can fit in to your hand) a day is the recommended minimum amount advised by the Food Standards Agency in the UK. However this is meagre compared to up to ten portions recommended in some other countries and most experts agree we should ideally eat more than five.

Beans and pulses count as a portion despite actually belonging to the protein food group. Fruit and vegetable juices can count for one small (150 ml) glass a day but anymore than this can't be counted. This is because juicing removes healthy fibre, and as it takes more than one fruit portion to make one glass, juices can be high in sugar and calories (See *Chapter 6, Liquid Energy*). Most fruit, vegetables and salad vegetables are bulky and low in calories so are a dieter's best friend. Watch out for avocados and olives which although are full of vitamins are also high in (healthy monounsaturated) fat so are higher in calories.

Frozen, tinned and dried fruit also all count as a portion and, although fresh is preferable, frozen fruit and vegetables can have as much if not more nutrients than fresh as freezing soon after picking locks in vitamins. Pre-cut vegetables lose their vitamins quickly, and in my opinion don't taste that great either, but can be useful occasionally if you are in a rush. Beware that removing water to dry fruit condenses it, making it higher in sugar and calories gram for gram, and the water soluble vitamins in the fruit are lost as well. The fresher the produce you can buy the better as it will not only retain more of its vitamins but will taste better too. Some supermarket produce can be days or weeks old so if you can get to a farmers' market or local farm shop it is worth the effort, but only in terms of quality and environmental consciousness – it won't have any bearing on the calorie content. Finally, you could grow your own vegetables – they do taste delicious, are an environmentally friendly way of eating, contain more vitamins and cost virtually nothing! But if gardening isn't you then that's fine, it's eating them in the first place which matters here so buy them from wherever is convenient if it helps you get your quota!

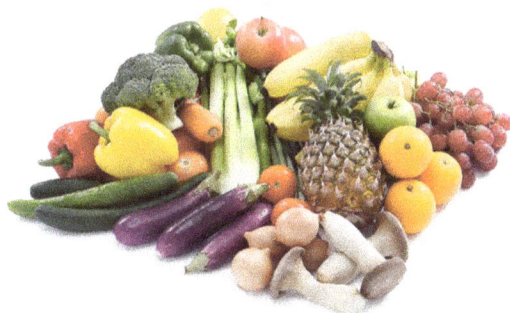

Buy one item of fruit or veg that you've never tried before each time you do your weekly food shop to stop boredom setting in. Make it a personal challenge to try every variety they sell!

A portion of fruit or vegetables is:
- 3 tbsp or 80 g vegetables
- Small bowl of salad
- 1 piece of fruit e.g. 1 apple, pear, orange
- 2–3 small fruits e.g. plums, satsumas
- 80 g berries or a handful of grapes
- 150 ml fruit juice (only one glass per day counts)

Dairy

For dairy products 2–3 portions a day is the recommended amount, a portion being 200 ml milk, 150 g yoghurt or 30 g cheese. These portions provide enough of the nutrients they supply such as calcium and vitamin D. Decreasing portions sizes will decrease your intake of these vital nutrients. However you can lower your calorie intake by choosing lower fat versions. Too little fat however will also inhibit nutrient absorption as some vitamins are fat soluble (see *Chapter 7, Where Do I Go From Here?*) making virtually fat-free food and drinks such as skimmed milk not necessarily the best choice. Dairy free alternatives such as soya or rice milk can be substituted for people with lactose intolerance, but make sure they are fortified with calcium, iron, and vitamins A, D, and preferably E and K as well. Supplements may be needed if you find it difficult to get these nutrients from elsewhere in your diet.

N.B. There has been a trend recently, especially in celebrity culture, to omit dairy in favour of soya and other alternatives (note the rise in sales of the soya latte etc), in the hope of improved health. People have been drinking cow's milk for thousands of years and it is still regarded as an important and healthy part of our diet, providing valuable nutrients including vitamins, fats, and protein. Cutting out dairy could prove inconvenient, expensive, awkward and not even healthier, so unless you have a diagnosed intolerance. (Always get confirmation with tests from a doctor or qualified dietician if an 'alternative' naturopath suggests you have an intolerance as while they can spot symptoms it cannot be confirmed without tests.)

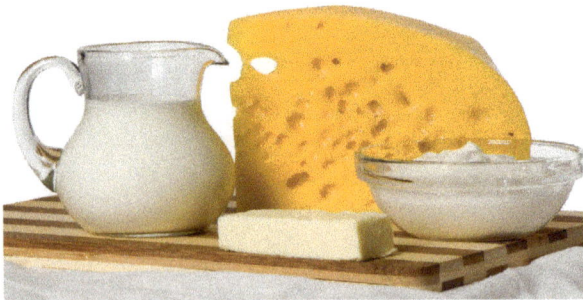

A portion of dairy is:
- 200ml milk
- Small pot (100–150 g) yoghurt, fromage frais, cottage cheese
- 30–40 g hard cheese e.g. Cheddar

Drinks

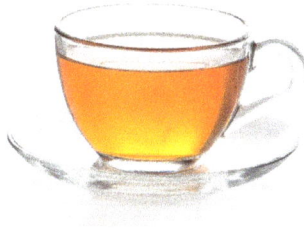

We should aim to drink eight glasses (2 litres) of fluid a day, more in hot weather or if exercising. Fruit juice, squash and milk count but aren't as thirst quenching as lower sugar drinks such as sugar free squash and diet drinks. Caffeinated drinks such as cola, coffee and tea also count but caffeine dehydrates in large quantities, so try to keep these drinks to a minimum. The best drink, of course, is water and you can liven it up with a slice of lemon or lime, or there are huge ranges of fruit or herbal teas available so if you've never tried them maybe give them a chance.

Alcohol

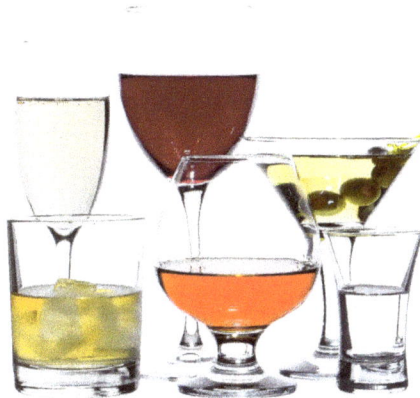

The recommended limits are 3–4 units per day for men and 2–3 per day for women, totalling 21 units for men or fourteen for women each week maximum. However it is good to have a couple of alcohol free days each week. The units in a drink depend on the percentage of alcohol and how big the serving is (drinks are given an 'alcohol by volume' percentage or ABV). A unit could be one 25 ml measure of spirits (40%), a third of a pint of beer (5–6%), or half a 'standard' 175 ml glass of red wine (12%). If you want to measure the units in your drink multiply the total volume of the drink (ml) by the alcohol ABV (%) then divide your total by 1,000.[15]

Calorie requirements

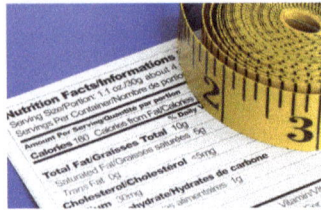

The average woman needs 2,000 calories a day to maintain a healthy weight, while the average man needs 2,500. However sedentary people such as those with office jobs may need less, while someone with a very active job or lifestyle may need more. Age also plays a part; young adults need more as they have a higher metabolism. A person's metabolism generally decreases with age. Metabolism is dependent on the presence of muscle, so you can keep a high metabolism as you get older by keeping your muscles strong and toned by doing weight-bearing exercise.

The number of portions you choose from each category will depend on your calorie requirements; if you need less calories you may choose two portions each of protein and dairy, for example, while if you need more you may eat three. So long as how many you choose is in proportion to the other food groups then your diet will be balanced.

80:20 rule

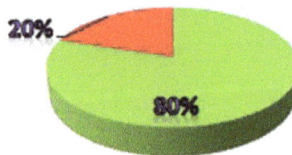

How well balanced your diet is will contribute to your overall health, as you will be getting all the nutrients your body needs to function at its best. However, as we have now established it is calories that count when it comes to weight. You could live on crisps or chocolate and not gain weight so long as you didn't consume more calories than you burnt off. However your overall health would be severely compromised. We could all eat the perfect diet all of the time, but then we'd miss out on treats such as cake and chips, and quite frankly life is too short! In my life aiming for 80 percent healthy with 20 percent treats (this is a maximum so don't feel you have to include treats if you would prefer to stick to healthier foods!) keeps the soul happy as well as the body healthy, and you should get enough nutrients while still enjoying the odd treat. The trick is to include these treats while not exceeding your calorie requirements and you won't gain weight.[3,23]

10 Feed Yourself Fuller

The British Nutrition Foundation (BNF)[22] has devised a good way of being able to eat a range of foods in the right proportions so that you don't gain excess weight, called the *Feed Yourself Fuller Chart*. It categorises foods according to their energy density, in other words the number of calories per gram. This chart is great for someone who needs to learn which are high and low calorie foods without having to memorise every numeric value of everything they eat as it categorises the foods into four easy to understand columns. The aim is to eat more low density foods, and less high density ones. However as the calorie values are given for a single gram, what you need to take into account is the real portion size that you would consume. For example, a 300 g bowl of very low density broccoli and Stilton soup would, according to the chart (0.5 calories/gram), have 150 calories. A 25 g bag of crisps on the other hand, would have only 133 calories, despite being in the high density column. The soup would be much more nutritious and filling so you are less likely to still feel hungry, but as far as losing weight is concerned, it's calories that count. However as the soup is more filling, you may not need anything else whereas after eating crisps you may still be hungry so snack on something extra, making your calorie intake higher in the end.

If you want to know more about the exact calorie content of different foods there are many 'calorie counter' books you can find in bookshops as well as websites that offer comprehensive listings that are often updated with new products. These usually show the calorie content for 100 g and also for a particular (and realistic) portion size to make it easier to calculate how much you are consuming.

If you only know the calories for 100g and want to work out the total calories for a portion of food, divide the calories per 100 g by 100, then multiply this figure by the total grams of what you are to eat. For example, if you were to eat 140g of Greek yoghurt from a large pot, at 145 calories per 100g:

(145/100) x 140 = 203 calories

Labelling of the nutritional value of food is quite commonplace on many products especially in supermarkets and mass-marketed products. However these can sometimes be the more processed products, so if you buy unlabelled food such as from farm shops and markets, a calorie reference book or a bit of knowledge can help you make the right choices.

British Nutrition Foundation *Feed Yourself Fuller* Chart

Very low energy density foods – go for it! You can eat big portions of these foods and use them to bulk out meals.

Low energy density foods – these foods make up most of what we eat and you can eat satisfying portions.

Medium energy density foods – it's especially important to eat oily fish like salmon, and to include lean sources of protein like steak, but you need to control the portion sizes of these foods and eat them alongside lots of lower energy density foods.

High energy density foods– these can be included in the diet, but in small portions or eaten less frequently. You can also try swapping them for lower energy density alternatives some of the time, for example, use a reduced fat spread instead of butter or margarine, try baked instead of standard crisps or a low fat soft cheese instead of hard cheese.

Energy Density kcal/g

Very	Low	Medium	High
Cucumber 0.10 Mixed salad 0.19 Chicken noodle soup 0.19 Broccoli 0.33 Carrots 0.35 Orange 0.37 Pear 0.40 Apple 0.47 Broccoli & stilton soup 0.50 Vegetable soup 0.52	Vegetable stir fry with noodles 0.63 Mixed berries with low fat yogurt, crunchy oat cereal & honey 0.71 Spaghetti Bolognese with lean mince, vegetables and whole wheat spaghetti 0.75 Low fat yogurt 0.78 Baked beans 0.81 Banana 0.95 Cornflakes with semi-skimmed milk 1.10 Baked potato 1.36 Boiled egg 1.47 Grilled chicken breast (without skin) 1.48	Strawberries and cream 1.6 Chocolate mousse 1.8 Spaghetti Bolognese with standard mince and cheese 1.9 Lasagne 1.9 Steak 1.9 Grilled salmon 2.2 Jam 2.6 Meat pizza 2.6 French fries 2.8 Croissant 3.7	Crackers 4.1 Regular hard cheese 4.2 Chocolate biscuit 4.9 Chocolate 5.2 Crisps 5.3 Roasted peanuts 6.0 Mayonnaise 6.9 Butter/margarine 7.4 Vegetable, olive or seed oils 8.9

The *Feed Yourself Fuller Chart* is created around the calorie content gram for gram of each food, and not nutritional content. Nuts, vegetable oils, cheese and salmon are highly nutritious and in the right amounts can contribute towards a healthy diet, despite being classed as medium and high density foods. Chicken noodle soup, whilst being low density (and therefore low in calories), could be low on vitamins and minerals if it were a processed, canned version, and could contain artificial additives and high levels of salt, making it not so healthy. For more details on what entails a healthy, nutritious diet, see *Chapter 9, A Balanced Diet*.

Real Meal Density Chart

This is my own reinvention of the chart, composed of popular foods in what I consider to be normal adult portions. Very low and low calorie items are good choices for snacks, whilst medium ones are better for meals, with high calorie meals saved as occasional treats. As with the BNF chart, this does not take into account nutritional content – something low calorie can be either very high or low in vitamins and other nutrients, and the same can be said of high calorie meals. You should still try to get all the nutrients you need to stay healthy, especially whilst cutting back on calories as there is more chance you could be deficient in certain nutrients if you are eating less food overall.

Very low (under 100 calories) – snacks that are under 100 calories should be easy to fit into any meal plan without overdoing the calorie intake over a whole day. High density foods will be quite small portions but fresh fruit and other low density choices are more satisfying. Two or three snacks throughout the day should be enough to keep you going if you are having a proper breakfast, lunch and supper.

Low (100-300 calories) – this would be a snack or very light meal. Try not to have more than two snacks from this group on top of proper meals or your total calorie intake will quickly add up. If you want more you may have to have smaller meals or cut back later.

Medium (300-500 calories) – most main meals will fall into this group and if breakfast, lunch and supper all add up to 1,500 calories then unless your calorie requirements are very low this still allows leeway for a couple of snacks in between.

High (500 calories or more) – it is important to enjoy whatever food you want to prevent getting depressed about having to lose weight, but keep these foods as treats or perhaps don't eat a whole portion. These foods are OK if you keep within your personal calorie needs most of the time, but if you like eating them more often you may have to cut back at other times to make up for the increase in calories.

Energy content of foods are estimated calories based on typical average recipes, as listed in the following table:

Very Low under 100 calories	Low 100–300 calories	Medium 300–500 calories	High 500 calories or more
Apple 60	Cereal bar 130	Small cheeseburger 350	½ a 10" thin crust margarita pizza 660
Digestive biscuit 70	Toast & 1 tsp butter & jam 200	200 g jacket potato with 200 g cauliflower cheese 400	400 g lasagne 500
Small banana 95	300 g minestrone soup 120	Large 75 g flapjack 350	Tuna Nicoise salad with dressing 550
Low fat instant chicken mug soup 89	Carrot sticks & a 50 g tbsp hummus 200	Ham & cheese toastie 450	300 g chicken and bacon pasta salad 650
Diet yoghurt 69	30 g of mixed nuts 195	3 egg cheese omelette 400	6 battered sweet & sour prawn balls 650
Peach 40	25 g bag of crisps 133	Large hot chocolate & whipped cream 350	Cornish pasty 550
1 rounded tsp butter 74	30 g Cheddar cheese 120	Prawn & mayo sandwich 370	Roast pork dinner with all the trimmings 800
Boiled egg 80	Cupcake 150	Pain au chocolate 300	Large thick strawberry milkshake 550
Meringue nest 55	Low fat chicken sandwich 280	50 g granola with a low fat yoghurt 360	400 g chicken curry and rice 630
Small skimmed latte 70	Strawberries & 50 ml cream 150	400 g spaghetti arrabiata 400	Club sandwich 650
120 ml glass of wine 92	45 g Cereal & semi-skimmed milk 250	Large fresh cream éclair 250	Banana split sundae 690
3 dried apricots 60	1 tbsp olive oil 135	400 g fish pie 400	Moules mariniere with chips 600
14 g mini box of raisins 45	250 ml Fruit & yoghurt smoothie 223	Slice of chocolate fudge cake 360	Chicken chow mein 570
2 multigrain crispbreads 80	Pint of beer 182	½ a garlic Baguette 350	400 g paella 540
Toasted crumpet 98	Small chocolate bar 140	400 g Lancashire hot pot 400	400 g beef stew and dumplings 600
Skinless chicken drumstick 90	Small tin of sardines 190	Individual spinach, tomato & ricotta filo tartlet 350	400 g mushroom Stroganoff and rice 540
Large slice of watermelon 80	330 ml can lemonade 140	120 g Cajun skinless chicken breast with 140 g potato wedges 300	Individual salmon en croute 500
3 Brazil nuts 90	Bagel & low fat cream cheese 270		
25 g plain popcorn 95	1 tbsp (60 g) coleslaw 150		
Mini doughnut 70			
Strawberry split ice lolly 75			
Small whole corn on the cob (no butter) 90			

So as you can see it is no use just categorising foods as healthy or unhealthy. Nuts are only fattening if you eat too many; half a 200 g snack pack of chocolate covered Brazil nuts would come to 607 calories! But Brazil nuts contain very healthy monounsaturated fats amongst other important nutrients such as selenium, and three whole ones are only 90 calories. Doughnuts are low in nutrients and have a high energy density as they are deep fried and covered in sugar, yet a mini one is only around 70 calories. 'Healthy' flapjacks may be full of nutritious oats and sometimes fruit and nuts too, but all that butter or oil, sugar and syrup make a modest shop bought 75 g single portion come in at 350 calories. A tuna Nicoise salad is packed full of nutritional foods; eggs, potatoes, tuna, fresh salad leaves and dressing with monounsaturated oils but an average portion could have 550 calories, with a restaurant serving more like 800.

It's not just what you eat that counts but importantly how much of it. Portion control is key when trying to cut calorie intake, as however 'fattening' or 'not fattening' you might think a food is, how much you eat of it is what dictates how many calories you consume. The chart above shows the calories in what I consider to be a reasonable 'normal' portion of each food. I hope that while reading this book you are learning that actually you can choose to eat whatever you like so long as you adjust the portion sizes or eat them less frequently. In the meantime, however, use the chart as a guide to help you choose the best snacks and meals for your needs.

11 Meal Examples

I expect you already know what constitutes a good balanced meal. On the other hand, you must be going wrong somewhere or you wouldn't be reading this book. It is easy to get stuck in a rut when it comes to deciding what to eat as it becomes so routine you could do the supermarket shop with your eyes shut. Embarking on a complete eating overhaul (unless extremely necessary for medical reasons) can be confusing and time consuming, so keep meals simple. Too much effort is one of the reasons people fall off the wagon from their strict self-imposed diets.

It is healthy to have a balanced combination of protein, carbohydrates, fruit or vegetables and fat at each meal. This will ensure you get a range of different nutrients, and have a range of flavours and textures to keep meals interesting. This is also the generic composition of most meals; spaghetti Bolognese, cereal with milk and a glass of juice, a ham and tomato sandwich and a roast dinner all conform to this structure.

Calories are not given for all meals in this chapter as some depend entirely on how much/what you choose, and others are estimates as recipes will all differ slightly, whilst branded products can vary slightly depending on which flavour you choose. I have included both homemade and bought foods and even fast food, proving that it is possible not to overeat whatever your food choices may be.

Breakfast

Not called the 'most important meal of the day' for nothing, breakfast kick starts your metabolism so you burn more energy throughout the day. People have been shown to perform much better, quicker and more efficiently after eating breakfast, whether at work, school, caring for children or whatever else fills your days. Interestingly studies show what you choose to eat doesn't make much difference to performance levels, so long as you eat something. However a balanced, wholesome, nutritious breakfast is going to give you more health benefits than a refined, sugary one. Here are some ideas whatever your morning preferences:

- 4–6 tbsp (or 45 g) cereal, 150 ml semi-skimmed milk, 125 g berries, glass of water or low calorie drink such as fruit or herbal tea (300 calories)
- two slices of toast topped with 1 tsp butter or spread and yeast extract, 200 ml glass of milk, a piece of fruit e.g. an apple (450 calories)
- a bread roll, one piece of lean back bacon (dry fried or grilled), sliced tomato, cup of tea (300 calories)
- a pain au chocolate and a bowl of fruit salad, small skimmed latte (450 calories)

- two eggs scrambled with 1 tsp butter, 1 piece of wholemeal toast, mushrooms and tomatoes, cup of tea (400 calories)
- two Quorn sausages, a medium bread roll, 100 ml fruit juice (350 calories)
- a piece of toast with 1 tsp each of peanut butter and jam, a piece of fruit, glass of water or fruit or herbal tea (350 calories)
- small cappuccino, an average fruit, nut and seed cereal bar, and a banana (300 calories)
- 150 g pot of full fat luxury yoghurt and large fruit salad, fruit or herbal tea (300 calories)

Lunch

Lunchtime is a chance to have a break, clear your head, and recharge your energy so that you can fully embrace the afternoon ahead. With that in mind it is helpful to choose foods that provide long lasting energy and prevent an afternoon 'slump'. Lunch can be homemade or bought, made of organic whole foods or processed fast food – which direction you take will impact your health and how you feel, but so long as you are not exceeding your personal calorie requirements you can, and should, stop to eat lunch. If possible a brisk walk in the fresh air before you eat will boost your metabolism and clear your mind (especially if you have spent the morning sitting down working), but whether at home or work, stop what task you are doing and try to sit down and relax to eat a proper meal:

- two slices of bread, 50–75 g of lean ham, beef, or turkey etc, 1 tbsp extra light mayonnaise, unlimited salad vegetables with fat free dressing, glass of water (350 calories)
- chicken burger from a fast food chain and a side salad without dressing, diet cola (415 calories)

Fresh soups (the chunky ones with lots of meat/veg/beans) are my emergency fallback and I always have a supply of them in my freezer. A whole tub is very filling and most are low calorie enough to eat the lot if you are hungry enough.

- 60 g grated half fat cheddar cheese on a piece of toast, grilled. 2 tbsp pickle and unlimited salad, glass of water (444 calories)
- two pieces of bread and 100 g low fat oven chips to make a low calorie chip butty! Serve with ketchup or extra light mayonnaise and unlimited salad, 100 ml orange juice (400 calories)
- jacket potato (200 g), a small (75 g) tin of tuna in brine or spring water, 2 tbsp extra light mayo, unlimited salad, glass of sugar free squash (350 calories)
- wholemeal pitta bread with 50 g reduced fat hummus, roasted peppers (roasted with spray oil or patted dry of any oily residue) and salad dressed with lemon juice and balsamic vinegar, fizzy water with lemon or lime wedge (350 calories)

Supper

Sometimes supper will be an enjoyable, leisurely, social gathering with family and friends. Other times it will be the quickest thing you can throw together as you stagger in the door after a long, tiring day at work. Neither situation has to be unhealthy or high calorie, expensive or boring, or take much time or effort. You just need to have a few things in the fridge, freezer and cupboard that you can rely on to form a meal that doesn't involve a large amount of calories:

- half a thin crust pizza with a side salad with light dressing, fizzy water with lime juice (approx 500 calories)
- two small low fat or Quorn sausages, 150 g mashed potato (made without butter), and unlimited broccoli and carrots, glass of water (400 calories)
- pasta with pesto (75 g dried pasta & 50 g pesto) & a large green salad, small glass of white wine (600 calories)
- two large fishcakes and unlimited vegetables, glass of water (450 calories)
- 75 g roast beef, one medium roast potato, one small Yorkshire pudding, two serving spoons of homemade gravy and unlimited vegetables, small glass of red wine (580 calories)
- Any 400 calorie ready meal with extra vegetables, glass of sugar free squash (450 calories)

See *Chapter 12, Home Cooking Tricks*, and *Chapter 16, Quick and Easy Meals*, for more ideas.

Pudding

Pudding is not a daily habit in our house but if I go to my Mum's for lunch I'll have a small portion (around a serving spoonful) of whatever she's made or bought (usually fruit crumble or a chocolate torte), or if I'm at a restaurant I'll have something light such as a sorbet or perhaps share with someone else as portions are usually large anyway. This is a good trick as you can have a taste of something delicious and indulgent as you like (chocolate melt in the middle puddings are a favourite in my group of friends!). The more calorific the pudding, the less you eat, and even just a mouthful can satisfy that desire to 'try' something that looks good on the menu. Then again if you want a fruit salad (minus the cream) then a whole bowl is still not going to add too many calories. At home, ice cream, sorbet, and individual pots of low fat yoghurt and mousse are easy and convenient.

Some ideas are:

- a pot of low fat mousse
  (60 calories)
- 75 g scoop of luxury ice cream
  (150 calories)
- two scoops of sorbet
  (110 calories)
- fruit salad or baked fruit
  (75 calories)
- sugar free jelly – I can't tell the difference from regular
  varieties (5 calories)
- one serving spoon of fruit crumble
  (150 calories)
- an eighth of an average fruit pie
  (220 calories)
- an eighth of an average chocolate torte
  (250 calories)

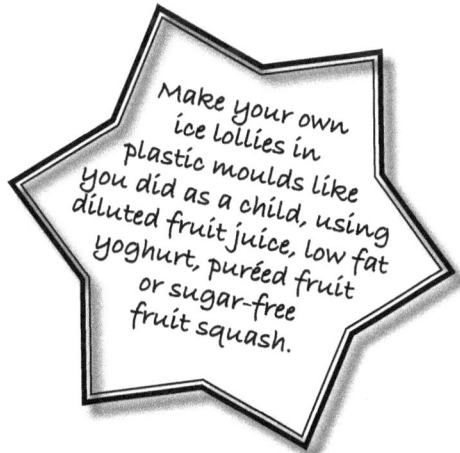

Make your own ice lollies in plastic moulds like you did as a child, using diluted fruit juice, low fat yoghurt, puréed fruit or sugar-free fruit squash.

Snacks

A couple of snacks a day is fine if it fits with the rest of your daily diet. Through reading earlier chapters I hope you have seen that no foods are forbidden, but only if you don't eat too much overall – you have to keep within your personal calorie needs.

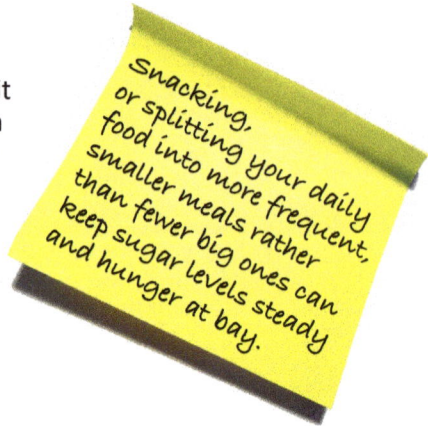

Snacking, or splitting your daily food into more frequent, smaller meals rather than fewer big ones can keep sugar levels steady and hunger at bay.

Here is a list of some fairly low calorie yummy treats which mean you won't be missing out – add fruit if you need something more filling:

- low fat ice cream stick (90 calories)
- snack size chocolate bars, or half a regular bar
- five whole raw brazil nuts (114 calories)
- 20 g bag of cheesy maize snacks (99 calories)
- small skimmed latte (102 calories)
- a banana (100 calories)
- cereal bar
- two chocolates from a sharing tin (100 calories)
- a small scone (200 calories)
- low fat hot chocolate sachet (40 calories each)
- 200 ml of warm semi-skimmed milk with vanilla extract – my nightcap! (100 calories)

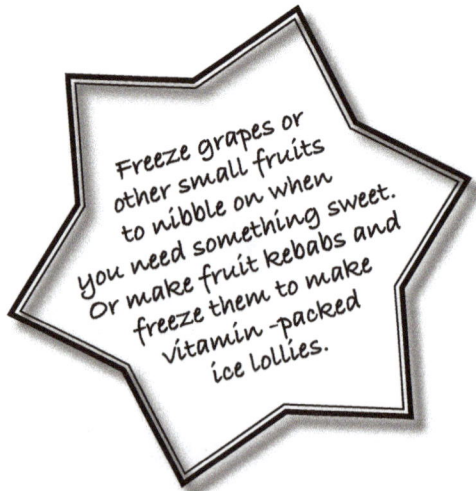

Freeze grapes or other small fruits to nibble on when you need something sweet. Or make fruit kebabs and freeze them to make vitamin-packed ice lollies.

12 Home Cooking Tricks

As I have said before this is not a recipe book so I have not included many. The next few chapters include simply a handful of examples of how usually high calorie meals can be made in more waist-friendly ways. I have tried to choose family favourites that you will find useful and will use often. I have also tried to pick meals that are traditionally very high in fat and calories because it is harder to find low calorie versions of these. I find it pointless when weight loss companies sell cookbooks and ready meals comprising of tomato sauces and lean meat for example, when these are already low in fat and calories; making 'diet' versions of these are easy and in my opinion a cop-out. What we all surely want is still to eat our favourite comfort food with the knowledge that we don't have to cut back on calories later or exercise to burn it off.

Here are the tricks you can use to cut calories in most meals. You will notice many of them in the recipes that follow. Try to apply these cooking tips to your own recipes, remembering to take into account portion sizes, which will determine the overall calorie content.

Spray oil
- Use spray oil which is only 1–5 calories per spray for:
  ▷ pan frying onions, mushrooms, eggs, white fish, shellfish, tofu, just about anything;
  ▷ greasing roasting pans and cake tins to help prevent food sticking while it cooks.

Ingredients that contain fat
- When cooking with ingredients that contain fat (e.g. mince or sausages) no oil is needed if you use a non-stick pan or baking dish, and drain any oil that comes out of the meat and pat dry with kitchen paper towel.
- Drain mince after browning before adding other ingredients.
- Drain meat for stir fries and casseroles before adding other ingredients.
- Dry fry or bake meat and oily fish.
- Fry onions, mushrooms and other vegetables in a non stick pan without oil, but use a lower heat and stir frequently to prevent them burning.

Thickening stews and sauces
- Instead of cream use cornflour or low fat crème fraiche to thicken:
  ▷ soups and casseroles;
  ▷ sauces for meat or pasta;

▷ any sauce or gravy that just needs thickening if it is too runny.

Cream

- Use low fat crème fraiche or fromage frais instead:
  - ▷ in puddings, for example with meringues in a Pavlova or Eton Mess;
  - ▷ as a cake topping or filling;
  - ▷ in anything which requires whipped cream.

Meat alternatives

Meat alternatives such as Quorn[24] can be significantly lower in fat and calories than meat, and are a good source of protein for vegetarians and meat eaters alike. Versions of most meat products from mince and chicken-style pieces to sausages and even Cornish pasties are available, and all can be used in your normal way, such as to make a Bolognese or casserole. They are not to everyone's taste and meat contains many beneficial nutrients, but as part of an overall varied diet, meat alternatives can be an easy way to cut calories.

- Use instead of mince, meatballs, casseroles and meat pieces in other dishes such as chicken in sauce with pasta.
- Replace sausages, bacon, hot dogs, burgers, paté, chicken nuggets, pies, pasties and ready meals – to name just a few.
- Meat can also be replaced (or use half and half) with lentils, chickpeas, beans and other pulses which are high in protein and fibre but low in fat and therefore lower in calories. As a bonus they also tend to be a lot cheaper than meat!
- Use half mince and half lentils in chilli con carne and use more beans.
- Replace some of the mince in Bolognese sauce with lentils.
- Replace some of the meat in a casserole with chickpeas.
- Use lentils, pearl barley or a pre-mixed 'soup mix' of pulses to thicken soups in place of meat.
- Blend cooked pulses with cream cheese and herbs to make a spread or pate.

Cheese

- Use strong cheeses such as mature Cheddar or parmesan as you need less to get the same flavour:
  - ▷ in cheese sauces for meat, fish and pasta;
  - ▷ to make cauliflower cheese;
  - ▷ mix with breadcrumbs to make a crust for meat, fish or as a pie topping;
  - ▷ to top pasta dishes and pies such as cottage pie;

▷ to add more flavour to soups;

▷ to sprinkle on salads.

Bulk up recipes

- Bulk up recipes such as stews with low calorie vegetables and use less meat:

  ▷ add grated carrot to bulk out mince in a Bolognese sauce and cottage pie;

  ▷ bulk out mince dishes with sliced onions, celery and mushrooms;

  ▷ replace some of the meat in stews and casseroles with chopped vegetables such as carrots, mushrooms, onions and leeks and celery.

Reduce fat

- Skim the visible fat which sits on the top of gravies, casseroles and sauces, like Bolognese, rather than stirring it in. Let them settle, then scoop up the oily residue floating on top. You can also use kitchen towel to soak it up.
- If eating later, once cold the fat will turn solid, making removing the layer of it sitting on top even easier.
- Trim visible fat off meat before you cook it, remove the skin from poultry and also trim the fat from ready cooked meats such as ham and leftover sliced roast meat before eating.

Low calorie, high flavour ingredients

Use herbs, garlic, sundried tomatoes, olives (in moderation due to the fat content), Worcester sauce, soy sauce and balsamic vinegar instead of butter, cream and cheese to flavour foods.

- Flavour a white sauce with parsley instead of cheese.
- Add a splash of Worcester sauce to Bolognese and beef casseroles.
- Fry mushrooms with garlic instead of lashings of butter.
- Soy sauce can be used as a salad dressing (with lemon or lime juice if you like), as well as to enhance Eastern dishes.
- Balsamic vinegar makes a good salad dressing on its own. It also goes well with tomatoes, peppers and other Mediterranean vegetables.
- Add chopped sun-dried tomatoes to salads, pasta or in sauces for chicken or fish for a strong hit of flavour, and add to tomato-based sauces to make them more intense.
- Olives and anchovies can be high in calories gram for gram when in oil, but as they are very strong in flavour you only use a very small amount. Pat dry of any residue oil with

kitchen paper then add to pasta or sauces for meat to make a simple but tasty dish.
- Marinating meat and fish in a sauce made from low calorie, high flavour ingredients for a few hours will make it tastier and more tender.

Avoid frying
- Grill, bake (without added fat), dry fry or stir fry (with little or no oil), or microwave instead of frying, and especially avoid deep-fat frying as food absorbs most oil this way.
- Grill meat so that the fat drips onto a tray or foil underneath.
- Dry fry meat and oily fish – the fat already present will stop it sticking.
- Microwave food to reheat it instead of frying. Stir it well halfway through and check it is hot all the way through with no burning hot or cold spots.
- Jacket potatoes and potato wedges can be precooked in the microwave to speed-up cooking time.
- Baking meat and fish requires no added fat as the meat uses its own juices; cover in foil to prevent drying out (remove for the last part of cooking), and pour away any oily liquid that seeps out from the meat.

13 Healthy, Tasty Recipes
Starters and Light Meals

If you are trying to cut the calories then having starters as well as a main course every day is really going to add up the calories and not help with weight loss. However on the odd occasion or when entertaining they are a way of showing your skill and generosity with food and make the meal last longer so you spend more time together round the table. Many traditional starters are deep fried (whitebait), cheesy (soufflé or fried Camembert), are covered in mayonnaise (prawn cocktail), or are naturally high in fat such as paté, so I have tried to find lower calorie recipes of popular starters so you don't have to resort to salad or carrot soup every time! These could also be light meals – just add a side salad and some bread for a lovely homemade lunch.

Cream of mushroom soup
Hearty doesn't need to be heavy – this soup is warm and satisfying without needing lashings of butter and cream.

Serves 8. 110 calories, 3 g fat per portion (240 calories, 16 g fat per typical portion made with cream)

Ingredients
- 4 leeks, white part only, chopped
- 3 finely chopped garlic cloves
- a small sweet onion, chopped
- pinch of salt
- pinch of freshly ground pepper
- 600 g fresh white mushrooms chopped
- 1 heaped tbsp plain flour
- 1.3 l chicken or vegetable stock
- 250 g reduced fat evaporated milk
- 1 rounded tbsp dried parsley

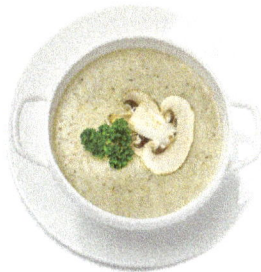

Method
1. Heat the oil over a medium heat in a large pot or saucepan, and throw in the leeks, garlic, and onion, stirring frequently until the leeks are soft (about 7 minutes).
2. Season with salt and pepper and add the mushrooms, cooking for a further 5 minutes.
3. Add the flour, stock, evaporated milk and parsley, and cook for another 10 minutes, stirring occasionally.
4. Leave to cook slightly before blending in a food processor or use a hand blender.
5. Reheat just before serving.

Chicken liver paté

Pate is normally made with the addition of animal fat (such as pork or duck), but this recipe shows it is not necessary, and paté lovers can still get their fix!

Serves 8. 90 calories, 5 g fat per portion (160 calories and 11.5 g fat per typical portion of Brussels paté)

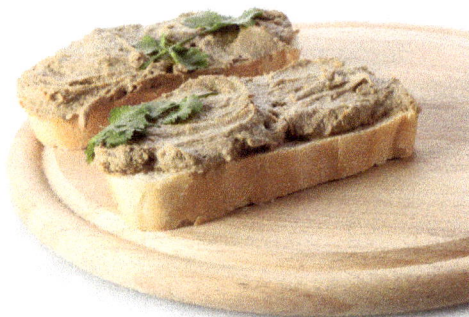

Ingredients
- 350 g chicken livers
- 3 cloves of garlic
- 20 g butter
- 1 medium onion, chopped
- 2 tablespoons of low fat crème fraiche
- 2 tsp brandy or sherry (optional)
- salt and ground black pepper

Method
1. Preheat oven to 200°c / Gas Mark 6. Place the chicken livers, butter, onion and garlic into an ovenproof dish and bake for 30 minutes.
2. Once the onion and garlic have softened, put the contents of the dish into a blender or food processor, then add the brandy, crème fraiche, some salt, and a little ground pepper, and blend until very smooth.
3. Spoon the mixture to a paté dish or other suitably sized dish and sprinkle with ground black pepper. Cover with cling film and chill in the refrigerator for a couple of hours.
4. Serve in slices with toast or for a lower calorie option salad (sliced radishes and rocket are good).

Baked sweet chilli filo prawns

A traditional favourite, baked instead of fried, with no additional oil needed.

Serves 8. 174 calories, 2 g fat per portion (360 calories and 25 g fat per typical portion)

Ingredients

- 8 thin sheets filo pastry (approx 250 mm²)
- 160 g sweet chilli sauce
- 160 g extra light mayonnaise
- 640 g cooked king prawns or tiger prawns (about 6 each), preferably with the tails on

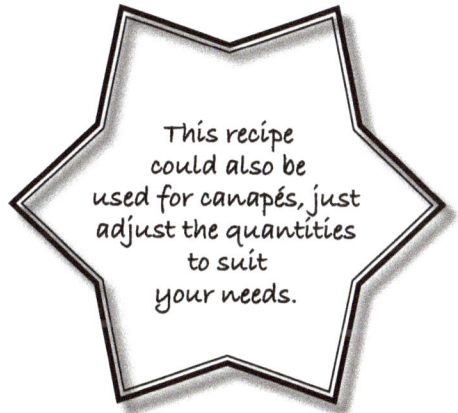

This recipe could also be used for canapés, just adjust the quantities to suit your needs.

Method

1. Cut each sheet of filo pastry into 6 strips, keeping the pastry you aren't using under a damp tea towel to avoid drying.
2. Brush both sides of the pastry strips with some sweet chilli sauce.
3. Wrap a strip of pastry around each prawn, leaving the tail exposed.
4. Place on a baking sheet and bake in the oven for about 4 minutes or until the pastry is golden brown.
5. Mix the remaining chilli sauce with the extra light mayonnaise and serve as a dip with the prawns.

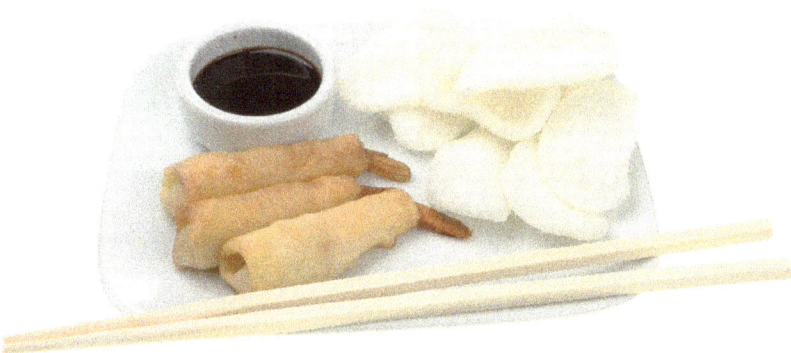

Nearly moules marinière

I call this 'nearly' as the original recipe requires butter and double cream. I have omitted both in favour of low fat and calorie fish stock.

Serves 4. 147 calories, 3 g fat per portion (390 calories and 11 g fat per typical portion of moules marinière)

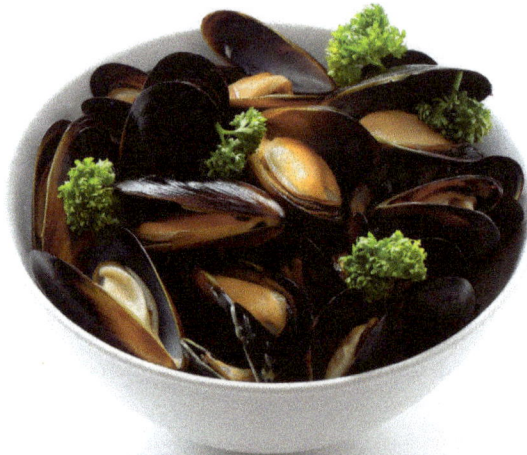

Ingredients

- 1 kg mussels (shell on)
- low calorie spray cooking oil
- 100 g shallots or small sweet onions, finely chopped
- 4 cloves garlic
- 125 ml dry white wine
- 150 ml fish stock
- 5 whole black peppercorns
- 1 lemon – juice and remaining halves of peel
- 3 tbsp fresh parsley, chopped

Method

1. Scrape and wash the mussels, removing the beard and any grit or sand, and throwing away any open mussels that don't close when you tap them, or ones with broken shells.
2. Fry the shallots using low calorie spray cooking oil until soft, then add the garlic and cook for a further 30 seconds.
3. Add the mussels, wine, stock, peppercorns, and lemon juice and peel halves and cover with a lid.
4. Cook on a high heat for 3 minutes or until the mussel shells have opened, throwing away ones that don't open.
5. Divide the mussels into four bowls and pour over the cooking liquid (leaving behind the lemon halves) and sprinkle with parsley.

Main Courses

A proper cooked meal is not something your Gran insisted on for no reason. A hearty meal consisting of cooked meat or fish (or alternative protein), some carbohydrates and plenty of vegetables provides a good portion of your daily nutritional needs, which is especially important if you are cutting your calorie intake. You are also less likely to snack later if you have eaten a proper meal.

Spaghetti carbonara

Sometimes only the full-fat, creamy version with buttery garlic bread on the side version will do, but to be able to enjoy it more often without the calories, this version comes close, Alpine views and ski boots optional! **Serves 4. 409 calories, 8.7 g fat per serving (traditional version 800 calories, 50 g fat per portion)**

Ingredients

- 3 big slices Parma ham or Serrano ham
- 1 tsp olive oil
- half an onion, chopped
- 2 cloves garlic, finely chopped
- handful fresh parsley
- 300 g (dry) spaghetti, preferably wholemeal
- 2 free-range eggs
- 2 tbsp half fat crème fraiche
- 4 tbsp Quark cheese
- 2 tbsp grated Parmesan cheese

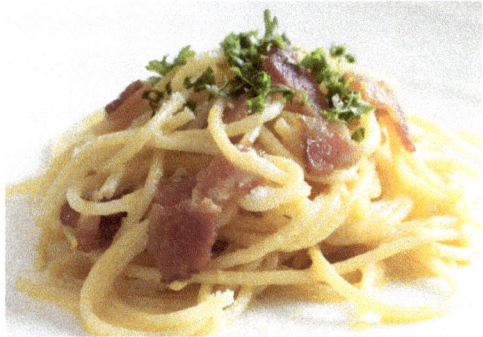

Method

1. Preheat the oven to 180°c / Gas Mark 4.
2. Place the Parma ham on a baking tray and bake for around 10 minutes until crisp.
3. Heat the olive oil in a large pan over medium heat and add the onion, garlic and parsley. Fry for 5–10 minutes until the mixture is soft and golden, then take off the heat.
4. Cook the pasta, then drain well and add to pan with onion mixture.
5. Whisk the eggs, crème fraiche and Quark together.
6. Add the mixture to the pasta in the pan, stirring until the mixture has cooked through.
7. Crumble the Parma ham into the pasta and garnish with Parmesan and some fresh parsley. Serve with a green salad or vegetables.

Chicken and broccoli pie

A family favourite which should keep everyone happy, whether watching their weight or not.

Serves 4. 376 calories, 18.5 g fat per portion (500 calories and 30 g fat per portion made with traditional shortcrust pastry)

Ingredients

- 2 skinless chicken breasts (about 300 g), cut into cubes
- 1 onion, diced
- 2 large carrots, chopped
- 1 broccoli (about 200 g), cut into florets)
- 170g (raw weight) filo pastry sheets
- 1 litre chicken stock (or 1 litre made with two stock cubes)
- 2 tbsp thyme
- 2 tsp olive oil
- 1 garlic clove, chopped
- 2 tsp cornflour
- 60 ml semi skimmed milk

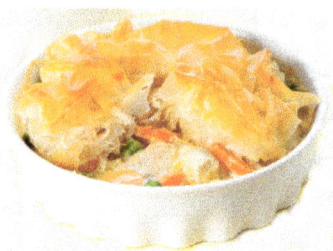

Method

1. Preheat the oven to 200°c / Gas Mark 6.
2. Heat the oil in a frying pan and fry the sliced chicken breasts until browned on both sides. Once cooked put in a 1.5 litre ovenproof dish.
3. Blanch the broccoli in boiling water for a couple of minutes, and add to the chicken.
4. Mix the cornflour with a little boiling water until it forms a paste, then add the milk.
5. Add the carrots, garlic and onions to the pan used for the chicken breasts and fry for 5 minutes until the onions are golden.
6. Add the stock to the pan and bring to the boil.
7. Once boiled add the milk and cornflour mixture then pour into the oven proof dish with the chicken and broccoli.
8. Add the thyme to the dish, then stir all the ingredients.
9. Scrunch the individual filo sheets on top of the chicken mixture so that the surface is covered.
10. Bake in the oven for about 50 minutes until cooked through and turning brown on top. Serve with extra vegetables.

Toad in the hole

Simple, quick and convenient, using mostly store cupboard ingredients and ideal for days when time is short and the fridge is bare!
Serves 4. 293 calories, 7 g fat per portion (480 calories, 16 g fat per portion of traditional version)

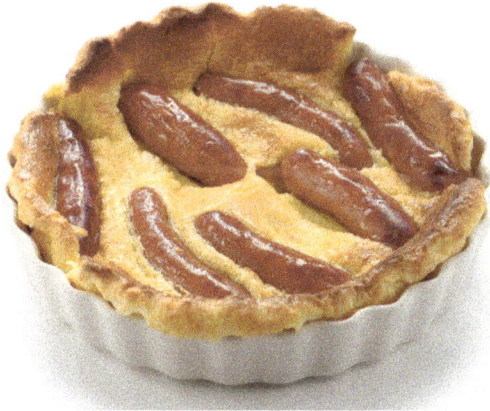

Ingredients

- 1 onion, cut into wedges and layers separated
- 8 thick low-fat pork sausages, or vegetarian sausages
- 1 tsp olive oil
- 100 g plain flour
- 1 free range egg
- 300 ml skimmed milk
- 2 tsp wholegrain mustard
- 1 tsp rosemary

Method

1. Preheat the oven to 200°c / Gas Mark 6.
2. Tip the onions into a small shallow non-stick tin (about 23x30 cm).
3. Arrange the sausages on top of the onions then add the oil and roast for 20 minutes.
4. Make the batter: sift the flour into a bowl, drop the egg in to the centre and beat in the milk a little at a time with a whisk, until it makes a smooth batter.
5. Stir in the mustard and rosemary and season with salt and pepper.
6. Pour the batter into the tin around the sausages and place in the oven for 40 minutes until the batter is risen and golden. Serve with steamed cabbage and carrots or swede, or tinned or frozen peas and sweetcorn if you've yet to get to the shops!

Vegetable korma

Making your own instead of a takeaway is both cost effective and could turn into part of the fun of 'curry night' with a group of friends. Don't be put off by the long list of ingredients; most are herbs and spices, which are useful store cupboard ingredients.

Serves 4. 362 calories, 13.4 g fat per portion, without rice (600 calories, 40 g fat in a typical vegetable korma)

Ingredients

- 1 kg mixed vegetables cut into small pieces (peas/beans, carrots, cabbage, squash, courgettes, aubergine, cauliflower, broccoli, mushrooms)
- 4 sprays of spray cooking oil
- 40 whole cashew nuts (about 40 g)
- 45 raisins (about 12 g), soak in water for a couple of hours
- 3 large onions
- 500 ml semi skimmed milk
- 4 tsp cornflour
- 3 tsp cumin seeds
- 4 tsp turmeric powder
- 6 tsp cumin powder
- 6 tsp coriander powder
- 2 tsp red chilli powder
- 4 tsp ginger-garlic paste
- 6 tsp garam masala
- 4 bay leaves
- a cinnamon stick
- 4 tbsp chopped fresh coriander

Method

1. Toast the cashews by frying in a pan without oil or on baking paper in an oven (200°C/Gas Mark 6) for 5–10 minutes until golden and set aside.
2. Heat a pan (or use the one used for toasting the nuts) and dry fry the onions.
3. Add a pinch of salt and the turmeric powder, red chilli powder, cumin powder and coriander powder, and stir often.
4. Blend the roasted nuts and onions in a food processor, adding a little water to form a thick paste.
5. Steam the cut vegetables (or microwave with a little water) until half cooked.
6. Heat the spray olive oil in the frying pan, add the cumin seeds and fry until brown.
7. Add the ginger-garlic paste and the nut-onion paste and stir fry for 1–2 minutes.
8. Add the cooked vegetables along with the water in which they cooked and the milk, and give everything a good stir.
9. Add a little boiling water to the cornflour to make a thick liquid and add to the pan, stirring until the mixture thickens.Add the bay leaf, cinnamon stick, raisins and garam masala and cook, covered, for 1 minute.
10. Stir in chopped fresh coriander and let the dish rest for 2–3 minutes.
11. Remove the whole bay leaves and cinnamon stick before serving.

Puddings

We all love pudding, and I mean proper ones not just low calorie fruit salad and yoghurts! Unfortunately they are not something you can gorge on if you want to lose weight. But with a few clever twists to recipes, you can make yummy favourites with far fewer calories so you can enjoy them occasionally without so much worry about what they are doing to your waistline. Especially good if you cook for a family who doesn't want to eat only 'diet food', as you can enjoy these as a treat together.

Chocolate cheesecake

Chocoholics are usually given two options: full fat or go without, especially in restaurants. If only there were more deliciously chocolaty low fat options such as this one.

Serves 12. 245 calories, 13.7 g fat per portion (450 calories and 30 g fat per typical portion of a traditional version)

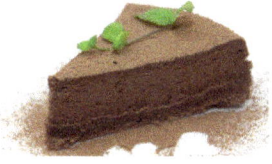

Ingredients

- 175 g reduced fat digestive biscuits
- 25 g cocoa powder
- 40 g reduced fat butter or spread, plus a little extra
- for greasing
- 150 g dark chocolate
- 3 free range eggs, separated
- 500 g ricotta cheese
- 150 g fat free crème fraiche
- 2 tsp cornflour
- 8 tbsp granulated sweetener
- 2 tsp vanilla extract

Method

1. Preheat the oven to 150°c / Gas Mark 2.
2. Grease the base of a 20 cm non-stick spring-bottom cake tin.
3. Crush the biscuits with the cocoa powder in a plastic bag with a rolling pin.
4. Melt the butter in a mixing bowl over a pan of hot water, and add the biscuit mix.
5. Press the mixture evenly over the base of the cake tin and refrigerate until set.
6. Melt the chocolate slowly in a small bowl over a pan of hot water and set aside to cool.
7. Whisk the egg whites until they form stiff peaks.
8. In a separate bowl, whisk the egg yolks, ricotta, crème fraiche, cornflour, sweetener and vanilla extract until smooth.
9. Whisk in the cooled melted chocolate to the mixture and fold in the egg whites.
10. Pour the cheesecake mixture over the biscuit base.
11. Bake in the oven for 50 minutes, and allow to chill before serving. Seasonal berries make a tasty and colourful accompaniment.

Bread and butter pudding

Comfort food at its best, without the calories it usually carries.
Serves 6. 236 calories, 5 g fat per portion (400 calories and 20 g fat per portion of a traditional recipe)

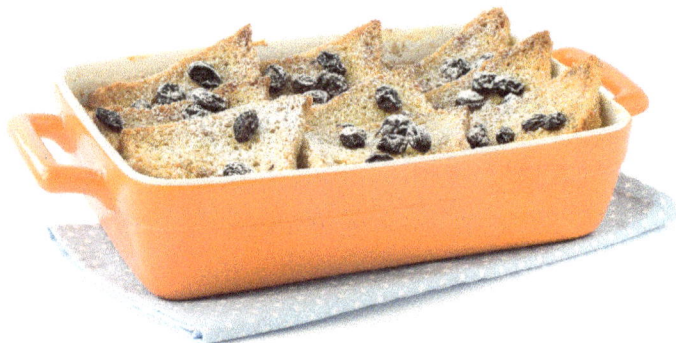

Ingredients

- 6 slices slightly stale bread (preferably wholemeal)
- 6 tsp very low fat spread
- 4 sprays low calorie cooking spray
- 75 g mixed peel, raisins or sultanas
- juice and grated zest of 1 medium orange
- 500 ml skimmed milk
- 3 tbsp (about 45 g) light brown sugar
- 2 medium free range eggs

Method

1. Spread the bread lightly with the low fat spread.
2. Spray a baking dish with the spray oil, and place half the bread in the bottom of the dish, spread side down.
3. Mix the peel with the orange zest and juice and spread over the bread.
4. Top with the remaining bread, spread side up.
5. Add the sugar to the milk and bring to the boil until the sugar has dissolved, then allow to cool for 5 minutes.
6. Beat the eggs in a large mixing bowl then add and stir in the warm milk.
7. Pour the mixture over the bread and fruit making sure no corners of bread have been left dry, and allow to soak for half an hour.
8. Preheat the oven to 190°c / Gas Mark 5.
9. Bake for 30–40 minutes or until risen with a golden crust.

Apple pie

A family favourite, with a recipe nobody will notice is low fat. Change the fruit to make it seasonal: pears, plums, rhubarb and cherries all work well.

Serves 8. 280 calories, 13 g fat per portion (506 calories and 29 g fat per portion of a traditional recipe)

Ingredients

Pastry
- 275 g plain flour
- 1 tsp salt
- 160 g reduced fat butter
- 2 tbsp golden or brown granulated sweetener
- 60–120 ml ice cold water

Filling
- 6 large (about 1kg total) Bramley apples; peeled, cored and thinly sliced.
- 4 tbsp golden or brown granulated sweetener
- ½ tsp cinnamon
- ¼ tsp nutmeg or mixed spice
- 1 tbsp lemon juice

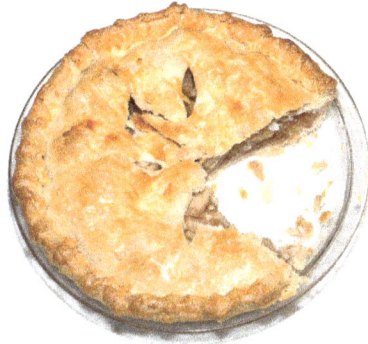

Method

1. Preheat the oven to 200°C / Gas Mark 6.
2. Sieve the flour and salt into a bowl, then add the sweetener.
3. Rub in the reduced fat butter until the mixture resembles fine breadcrumbs.
4. Gradually add the cold water to the dough, kneading and mixing until evenly coloured and textured, and the right consistency to roll out (like play dough).
5. Mix the sweetener with the nutmeg or mixed spice and cinnamon.
6. Divide the pastry in half, and roll out one half big enough to line a 20 cm tin or pie dish, trimming the excess pastry round the edges with a knife.
7. Lay the sliced apples over the pastry, drizzle over the lemon juice, and sprinkle over the sweetener and spices.
8. Roll out the remaining half of the pastry, moisten the edges with water, then place, moist edges down, on top of the apples.
9. Press down the edges of the pastry to make sure they are sealed, then prick the middle with a fork.
10. Bake for 20–30 minutes until the pastry is golden brown, and serve either hot or cold.

Tiramisu

A retro dinner party favourite, this is impressively tasty and sophisticated yet surprisingly simple to make.

Serves 6. 248 calories, 2 g fat per portion (450 calories and 35 g fat per portion of a traditional recipe)

Ingredients

- 12 trifle sponges
- 2 tbsp instant espresso coffee powder
- 3 tbsp Tia Maria
- 750 g Quark cheese
- 3 tbsp brown or golden granulated sweetener
- 2 tsp vanilla extract
- 3 tsp cocoa powder

Method

1. Cut the sponges in half to resemble fingers, and lay half of them in a deep glass serving dish.
2. Mix the coffee powder with 2 tbsp hot water, then stir in the Tia Maria, and pour half over the sponge in the dish.
3. Mix the Quark, sweetener and vanilla, and spread half over the soaked coffee sponge in the dish.
4. Layer the remaining sponges on top of the Quark, pour the remaining coffee mixture over, and top with the remaining Quark mixture. Chill for at least 2 hours, or overnight.
5. Sieve the cocoa powder over the Tiramisu before serving.

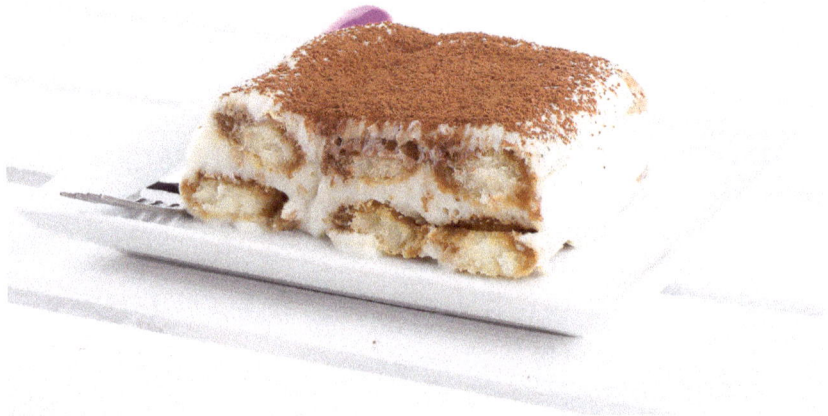

Sugar free courgette cupcakes

If you've not tried using vegetables in cakes before I highly recommend it, as it keeps the cakes moist so you don't need so much added butter or oil. **Serves 20. 107 calories, 3 g fat per portion (305 calories and 16 g fat for a typical iced cupcake)**

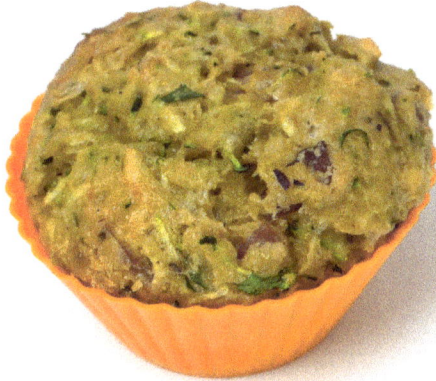

Ingredients

- 100 g reduced fat butter or spread
- 300 g plain flour
- 2 tsp bicarbonate of soda
- 200 g sugar free apricot jam
- 500 g grated courgette (including peel)
- 1 tsp vanilla essence
- 100 ml semi skimmed milk
- 2 tsp ground mixed spice

Method

1. Preheat the oven to 180°c / Gas Mark 4.
2. Cream the butter with the jam in a large bowl until light and fluffy.
3. Add the vanilla essence and milk and stir well.
4. Stir the courgettes into the mixture.
5. Add the bicarbonate of soda and mix thoroughly.
6. Spoon into cupcake cases and bake for 20 minutes or until risen and starting to go golden on top.
7. Sprinkle the mixed spice on top of the cupcakes and serve either warm or cold.

Quick and Easy Meals

Perfect fast food to knock up for one, two, or indeed a whole family! You can vary the ingredients and quantities slightly, it won't make much difference, but can be useful as you can just use whatever you have in the fridge or cupboard instead of having to go to the shops. Just make sure you always choose lean and low fat versions where possible.

English fry up

Serves 1

427 calories and 11 g fat per portion

Grill two lean turkey rashers and one lean low fat sausage, a handful of mushrooms and a tomato, cut in half. Meanwhile in a non-stick pan dry fry a medium free range egg, and slowly heat up 1/4 can (about 100 g) baked beans. Serve all of the above on a slice of wholemeal toast.

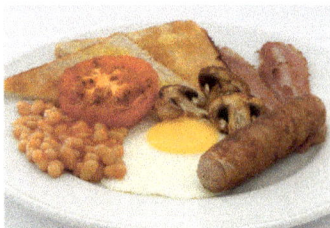

Boston beans

Serves 2

364 calories and 5 g fat per portion

In a non-stick pan dry fry a sliced medium onion and two rashers of lean back bacon (sliced widthways into strips). When cooked, add a 400 g can of baked beans, a dash of Worcester sauce, and some ground black pepper. Heat through, stirring continuously. Meanwhile toast two wholemeal muffins. Serve the beans on the hot muffins. Serve with grilled tomatoes and mushrooms if you are extra hungry.

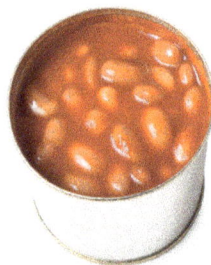

Tuna melt

Serves 1

398 calories and 13 g fat per portion

Drain a small (80 g) can of tuna in spring water or brine, and mix with 2 tbsp very light mayonnaise. Split a small (individual, around 65 g) ciabatta loaf in half, and put under the grill (outside facing up) to toast. When toasted spread the tuna mix onto the inside (untoasted side) and sprinkle with 30 g Emmental cheese, and

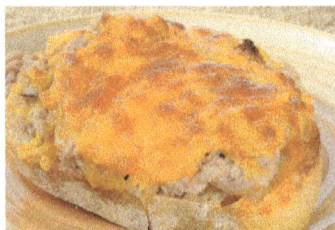

put back under the grill until the cheese melts. Serve with a green salad and sliced tomatoes drizzled with oil free Italian style dressing.

Potato wedges

Serves 1
353 calories and 9 g fat per portion

Cut a 200 g jacket potato into eight wedges and microwave on full power in a suitable dish with ½ cm of water in the bottom for about 3–4 minutes (or until edibly soft but not mushy. Transfer to a small roasting tin or baking tray lined with baking paper and put under a preheated grill for a couple of minutes until the wedges start to crisp slightly. Meanwhile dry fry 80 g mushrooms. Top the wedges with the mushrooms, 50 g shredded wafer thin ham, and 30 g grated reduced fat Cheddar cheese. Return to the grill until the cheese has melted, and serve with a green salad.

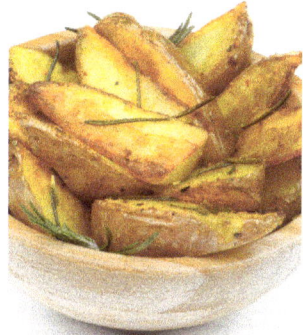

Spanish omelette

Serves 1
305 calories and 15 g fat per portion

Heat four sprays of calorie controlled spray cooking oil in a small frying pan and fry half a chopped onion. Meanwhile boil or microwave 100 g sliced or chopped potato (small waxy ones are ideal but not essential) then add to the pan. Pour over two beaten medium free range eggs and allow to cook through slowly on the lowest heat setting. Turn out onto a plate and serve with a green salad and chopped mixed peppers.

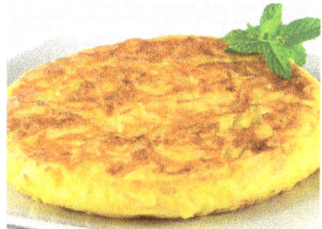

Mummy's mushroom pasta

Serves 2
311 calories and 4 g fat per portion

Boil 100 g (dry weight) pasta, preferably wholemeal. When cooked, drain and stir in a 295 g can of low fat condensed mushroom soup and a drained 200 g can of sweetcorn (about 165 g drained). Heat through and serve with steamed broccoli.

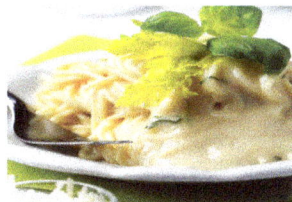

99

Vegetable soup

Serves 2–4
75 calories and 2 g fat for a quarter of a typical recipe without bread.

Chop 1 kg whatever vegetables you have to hand and put in a large saucepan with 1 litre vegetable or chicken stock (typically two stock cubes). You can use any vegetables but potatoes and parsnips do contain slightly more calories; other hearty root vegetables such as butternut squash, swede and carrots are also good 'thickeners' but are lower calorie. Onions, leeks and celery add lots of flavour. Serve straight away or reheat later, either as a low calorie starter or with rustic wholemeal bread as a light meal.

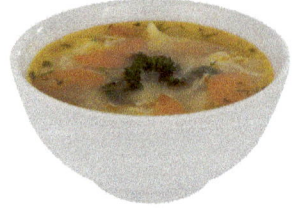

Eton mess

Serves 2
158 calories and 6 g fat per portion

In a bowl mix together 75 g each of low fat fromage frais and low fat crème fraiche. Roughly break two readymade meringue nests (about 14 g each) into the bowl and stir gently. Roughly chop 160 g strawberries (mash a few with a fork if you like) and stir into the mix. Serve straight away to prevent the meringues going mushy.

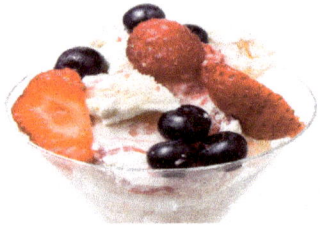

For an even easier and lower calorie version replace the fromage frais and crème fraiche with fat free Greek yoghurt, making the total calories 118 per portion

Chocolate ice cream sandwich

Serves 1
210 calories and 7 g fat per portion

Put a 40 g scoop of low fat chocolate or vanilla ice cream between two reduced fat chocolate digestives so that the chocolate coated sides are facing into the ice cream. Wrap in cling film and squash down slightly so that the ice cream is held tighter and evenly spread between the biscuits, and return to the freezer to set hard for fifteen minutes before eating.

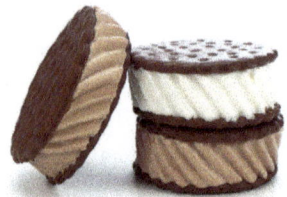

14 The Diet Plate

Kay Illingworth invented The Diet Plate® in 1995 – the world's first portion control plate. She works in conjunction with Dr Ian Campbell MBE, founder of the National Obesity Forum and medical adviser to Kay's company, Perfect Portion Control Ltd.

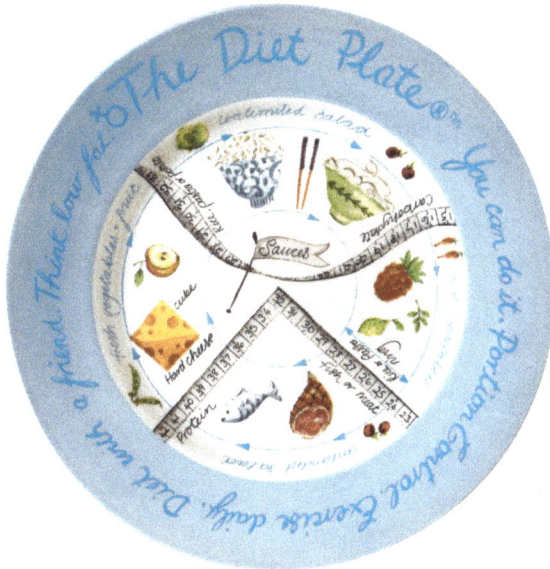

See www.thedietplate.com for more information and how to purchase the plate

The concept is simple: you use the guidelines and pictures on the plate (there is also a bowl version for soup and cereal, and different plates for male or female requirements), to show you how much of each food group is the correct amount for a balanced diet. Not exceeding the recommended portions restricts calories to some degree whatever foods you choose, though of course choices lower in fat and less 'dense' in calories will have a lower overall calorie content than the same size portion of calorie dense foods.

This method is ideal for anyone reluctant to count calories or with limited dietary knowledge as the plate does the work for you. The female one delivers 1,200–1,500 calories per day and the male 1,500-1,900 calories a day, which will deliver an average weight loss of 2.2lbs a week. Clinical trials[25] concluded that those who used the Diet Plate 80% of the time, were six times more likely to lose weight, as well as three times more likely to control blood sugars and lose more than 5% of body weight in a six month period.

15 Anywhere, Anytime

The great thing about eating 'normally' is that there is no excuse not to as you can do it anywhere. In almost any situation you can have a balanced meal. In fact the times you can't are so far and few between that they should have no effect on your weight (I can't actually think of any times because if in doubt just eat less of any calorie dense foods on offer). One meal, or even one day won't make a difference if you eat healthily most of the time. Below are a few examples where you may have thought eating healthily was impossible. I'm not implying these meals are the best choices for supplying nutrients and contributing to health but if you choose the right dishes you are at least making some difference.

Of course you can order whatever you wish but only eat a little of each, but be aware that calorie dense foods will require you to eat much smaller portions so you may feel less satisfied if you can't fill up on low calorie foods alongside (such as adding an undressed salad). Alternatively, you could eat until your heart's content but eat less for the next few days to balance it out. In all cases it is necessary to watch portion sizes as even low calorie foods are fattening if you eat too much of them.

Burger bar

The calories and fat in burgers varies between each restaurant, but some choices are easier such as having a regular (or kid's if possible) size burger rather than a quarter pounder. Skip the cheese and bacon and maybe add mushrooms, which even fried, are not so calorific so can be added without too much worry. Chicken, vegetable and bean burgers are not necessarily lower in calories. Choose a bun or chips (you only need one sort of carbohydrate) and add a side salad, being mindful of dressing (asking for it on the side gives you the option of adding as much or little as you choose). Mayonnaise is a common culprit with this sort of meal so you can ask to have it made without, but tomato ketchup, while not being entirely healthy and can be very high in salt, is actually quite low in calories.

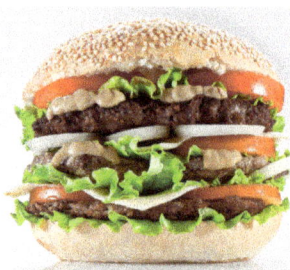

Chinese

A tough one as most Chinese foods, even vegetables, are fried and come in sweet sauces. Stir fried vegetables are a good option and most sauces with vegetables are fairly light although sweet and sour or satay sauces

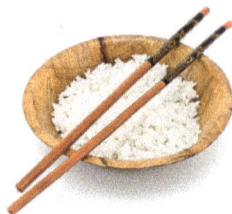

are more calorific. Anything in batter or deep fried is best avoided. Fish and chicken are usually lower calorie than beef, pork and especially duck but this does depend on how lean it is and how it is served. Boiled or steamed rice rather than fried is obvious. Chinese soups are quite watery which makes them less dense in calories. Chop suey is lower calorie than chow mein as the meat is served with bean sprouts rather than noodles. A meal of chicken with mushrooms, boiled rice and mixed chinese vegetables could potentially be quite a balanced meal and will not pile on the pounds so long as portion sizes are not too big.

Don't feel you have to order rice or noodles just because everyone else does. Have some stir fried vegetables along with a main, or share a rice dish with a friend as portions are usually large.

Fish and chips

Virtually everything from a chippy is deep fried, except for sides such as baked beans, mushy peas (the lowest fat options), and coleslaw. This makes them much higher in fat and calories than if you were oven cooking the same foods at home. Also the cooking oil is used over and over again which makes it very high in trans-fatty acids (see *Chapter 9, A Balanced Diet*).

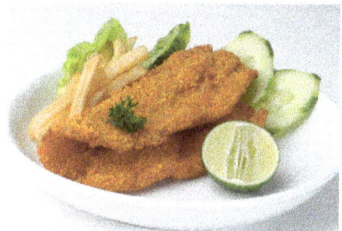

Breaded fish is a lower calorie alternative option to batter if it is available. A fishcake comes in at 230 calories compared to 295 calories for a small cod portion, the small difference mostly due to the smaller portion size. Some takeaways offer child-size portions, and you could add a salad or some fruit after if you are still hungry. Even a 'small' portion of chips could be up to 400 calories so best to have just a couple of someone else's to avoid calorie overload, or skip the fish and have just chips but as fish is much higher in protein than chips it will be much more filling.

Chips and cheese is a more recent addition to a chippy's menu but is a dieter's nightmare at 800 calories for a portion, and a quarter of a portion (a reasonable 200 calories) is going to be so small on your plate you'd be very hungry if you didn't fill up on salad alongside. And watch the little extras – mayonnaise is much higher in fat and calories than ketchup or vinegar (which is virtually calorie free), while gherkins are only five calories each but a pickled egg is about 90 calories, the same as a boiled egg.[22]

Indian

Plain or marinated meat such as tandoori or tikka have less fat and more hunger-satisfying protein than creamy sauces such as korma. Boiled or steamed

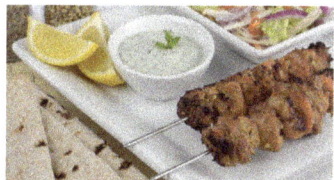

rice has fewer calories than pilau or fried rice. Vegetable side dishes can add calories if they are cooked in a creamy or greasy sauce, and many Indian restaurants do side salads so it's worth asking even if it's not on the menu. Nan bread and poppadoms, as another carbohydrate, are best avoided unless you want to have them instead of rice, though at around 40 calories for a small poppadom, one is not going to hurt.

Italian

Pasta can be high or low density calories depending on the sauce – creamy or meat sauces being much more calorific than tomato or vegetable-based ones. Usually the reputably high calorie content of pasta dishes is due to large portion sizes, so eat less and add a salad to fill you up. Garlic bread is high in calories, but olives are only five to ten calories each.

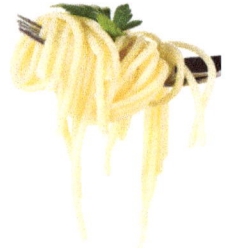

Kebab house

Döner kebabs are made from minced meat and often a variety of meats are used all at once. Mincing can also disguise poor cuts of meat, fat and connective tissue, and these are generally an unhealthy choice. Much better is a shish kebab of cubed meat, so not only can you see exactly what you are getting but even fried versions are likely to be better than a döner. Choose salad over chips, and although chilli sauce will not be high in calories, garlic or other creamy sauces may be based on mayonnaise or full fat yoghurt so you may want to stay clear of these.

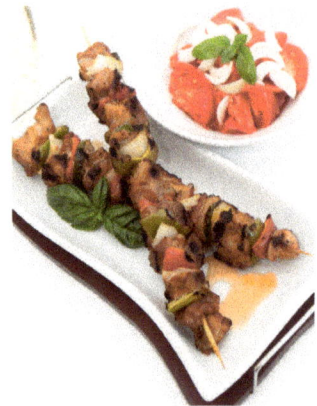

Pizza

A whole pizza can be quite calorific, so try a half with a side salad. Some well- known restaurants even offer to put different toppings on each half so you can share with a friend. Thin crust are much less fattening than deep pan purely due to the size, so an alternative might be a quarter (or one slice depending on the pizza's diameter) of deep pan pizza with salad. Beware the cheesy filled crust varieties – all that extra cheese is extra calories.

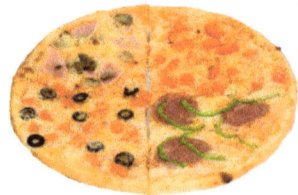

Christmas

According to the British Heart Foundation[1] the average person consumes 7,000 calories on Christmas Day! No wonder people put on an average of 5 lb over the festive season as this doesn't take into account all the extra party nibbles, drinks and mince pies in the weeks before and after the day itself. But it doesn't have to be this way. No one wants to miss out, and only a humbug would abstain from enjoying all the treats on offer at this time – a person more preoccupied with dieting than Christmas is not one I'd want at my party! The trick here is to have a little of everything you fancy, and then you won't feel like you are missing out as sometimes a taste is all you need. The party season covers a broad spectrum of situations so I have divided it into sections:

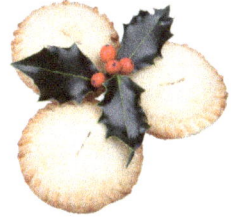

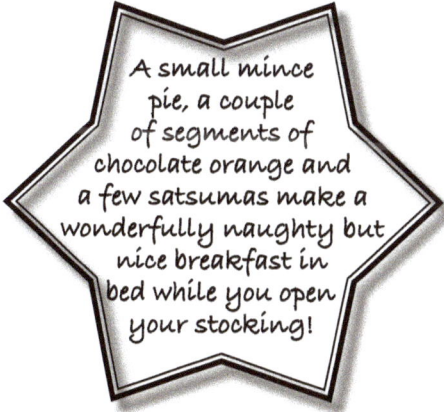

> A small mince pie, a couple of segments of chocolate orange and a few satsumas make a wonderfully naughty but nice breakfast in bed while you open your stocking!

Buffet

Anything with pastry is going to be high fat and therefore calorie dense. Sandwiches can vary depending on the filling and how much butter or mayonnaise is used (usually a lot in my experience, and caterers rarely use reduced fat versions). Lean protein such as skinless chicken legs (feel free to remove the skin yourself) will fill you up, but beware that most party meats such as sausages, mini kebabs and scotch eggs are processed and are dense in calories . Undressed salads are obviously the lowest calorie choice if available, which they often aren't! In a buffet situation the best you can probably do is to choose a few of whichever items you fancy but only to fill half a plate; probably three to five items depending on their size and how calorie dense they are. Fill up on salad if possible or have some fruit or vegetable soup when you get home to fill the gap. However, as high fat foods are more satisfying in smaller amounts than fat free foods, you may not feel hungry, especially with the distraction of people to talk to at a party.

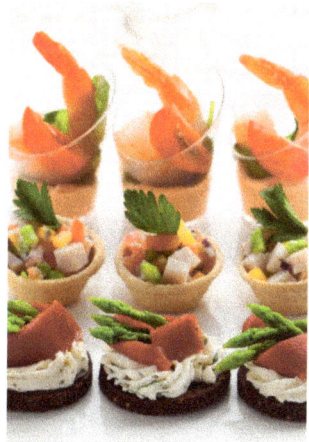

Nibbles

If it is not a mealtime, do you need extra snacks? Are you really hungry? If it will be a while until the next meal have just enough to keep you going – bear in mind this may only be a couple of crisps, you can always have a couple more later if you are still hungry. Nuts are more filling (and contain healthy fats) but are just as calorific as crisps. Dips vary from high calorie (creamy or oily ones such as taramasalata, guacamole, hummus and smoked fish pates) to less calorific (tomato or salsa ones). Mince pies and chocolate can be eaten in the same way you might have a mid-afternoon snack; one mince pie is around 200 calories, three chocolates around 150 calories, and a small (60 g) slice of Christmas cake 220 calories. Just make sure you choose only one, not all three options!

Christmas lunch

The 'little of everything' method is necessary to keep calories down as a traditional Christmas lunch is much more than a simple meat and two veg, where you could afford larger portions of each. Try one of everything – a small slice of turkey (or nut roast), one roast potato, one stuffing ball, one chipolata in bacon, and a tablespoon of bread sauce. Where you can indulge, of course, is the vegetables, but beware of how they are prepared such as caramelized with butter and sugar, or with diced bacon and chestnuts, as this will up the calories. Gravy made from granules is quite low calorie whereas when made from meat juices it contains more fat. In either case it should compliment your food not drown it!

Have a small portion of pudding with a serving spoon of custard or brandy sauce. Brandy butter is so calorific (simply sugar, butter and brandy) at around 100 calories for a rounded teaspoon it is not a 'dieter's friend' but as it's only once a year, a little of what you fancy will do the soul good!

Anywhere

You can always ask for dressing or sauces on the side, no butter or oil on vegetables or bread, and cut out or swap bits of a meal altogether (for example, extra vegetables instead of creamy potato dauphinoise) if you think you will be too tempted to eat the lot. Watch the calories you drink – wine, beer, fruit juice and fizzy drinks are the most commonly consumed when eating out but you don't have to follow the crowd. Swap sugary fizzy drinks for diet versions, have a spritzer (wine diluted with fizzy water) instead of wine, and if you choose fruit juice try to make it just one small glass.

Puddings don't have to be excluded. A fruit salad (minus the cream) is a very waistline-friendly option. Sorbets can be quite low calorie at around 55 calories per scoop. One scoop of average ice cream will come in at around 100 calories but luxury fresh cream ones will be more. If you just want a taste of something yummy why not share with a friend then only eat a couple of mouthfuls, or maybe have a taste of someone else's (but perhaps restrict this to close friends or relatives to avoid seeming rude!). Fruit puddings are not always healthier – apple crumble is fairly calorific and can be up to 600 calories for a hefty restaurant portion. Canned 'squirty' aerosol cream is surprisingly the lowest calorie choice at 50 calories for a 12 g serving, due to the fact that the cream is pumped with air so you don't use as much. Custard comes in second at around 100 calories/100 g, then single cream at 200 calories/100 ml. So the higher the calorie content, the less you should have.

Ask for child or starter size portions of main meals if you think you won't be able to stop yourself eating all of a large plateful.

Conclusion

I firmly believe eating out and social occasions are not an excuse for overeating or putting on weight, as even if you do overindulge there's nothing to stop you cutting back slightly the rest of the day or even exercising later in the week to make up for it. Socialising around food is great fun and important for bonding with friends and building relationships. I have often heard people with jobs that require lots of entertaining and eating out blame this for their weight problems, but as you can see there is no reason it can't be done regularly whilst staying healthy if you make the right choices.

Not sure whether you are really hungry? Have a (low calorie) drink then wait twenty minutes to see if you still want something to eat.

16 Learn to Listen

This is a skill which will have to be relearnt if you have lost your ability to use food purely to fuel your body. The very reason most people have weight problems is because they have lost touch with the instinctive reasons we need to eat in the first place; to satisfy hunger and sustain a healthy body.

Babies and young children can be notoriously picky eaters. Granted, sometimes toddlers are stubborn and use food as a way of getting attention or gaining control over their parents, but I think they have also yet to lose touch with their appetite, and eat simply because they are hungry. They won't always finish their plate, sometimes they won't have a bite, and other times they'll want third helpings! This is classic behaviour from my daughter, yet she is average height (despite me being short), a healthy weight, very rarely gets ill, and has boundless energy. So I trust that she knows how much to eat and don't push her as I want her to stay in touch with what her body is telling her. I do make sure that what she eats is a healthy, balanced and varied diet, but even then she has some days when she chooses mostly carbohydrates and other days when protein is preferable, and others when she'll happily eat fruit all day. It all balances out in the end. I don't think a little bit of hunger – waiting fifteen minutes for supper to be ready rather than having a biscuit in the interim for example – does her any harm, but what it does mean is that she finishes the healthy meal I've cooked her instead of half of it ending up in the bin.

If we could re-educate our minds and bodies to follow our intuitive physical needs when it comes to eating we would all be very healthy. Your body is clever; it knows what it needs and will tell you. For example, you probably understand that when you are extremely thirsty you get a dry mouth and a headache if you are too dehydrated – and you can respond accordingly with a drink. But as a nation we have largely lost our ability to tell the difference between physical hunger and emotional hunger or boredom, and more specifically what it is we need if we are hungry. Your body knows what it needs which is why you crave it. The exception here is fatty and sugary foods which, when eaten, will make you crave more of these types of foods without actually needing more, and this is why junk food is so appealing and comforting. Some women find they crave iron-rich foods such as red meat, baked beans and chocolate when menstruating. Along with their instinctive appetite needs that I talked about above, babies and young toddlers, left to choose their own food, have been found to choose more protein after being ill and more carbohydrate when they are having a growth spurt[27]. As I have stated numerous times, if you give your body what it is asking for, it should not ask you for any more.

I do believe that whilst some cravings are out of addiction such as is often the case with sugar, sometimes it is a need for certain nutrients.

Sometimes the reasons are quite clear cut – it is suggested that the cravings women experience during pregnancy are due to the need for specific vitamins and minerals. I always try to listen to my body and satisfy those cravings for fattening foods by finding a low calorie alternative. For instance if I am craving chocolate, it could be sugar I am craving, in which case fruit would satisfy, or else could it be a caffeine hit? If so, a coffee would do. If I fancy chips, carbohydrate rich toast or oatcakes will usually hit the spot. Or for ice cream, a vanilla or toffee-flavoured low fat yoghurt can be a good substitute. Not quite as good as the real thing, but my point is that my body was clearly asking for certain nutrients, so by eating these food types without consuming too many calories, I kept the cravings at bay. If you can learn to tune into your body you can give it everything it needs, be it carbohydrates, proteins, or simply a drink of water. Pause before grabbing something to eat or drink and take a moment to contemplate what it is you really want, as in what type of food it is (dairy, carbohydrates etc), then try to think of something healthy that would fit into these categories. You should not feel deprived if your body is getting all it needs, but if you have a large appetite then fruit is a high fibre, high water content, low calorie snack that is also contains lots of vitamins, and you'd have to eat a lot (not easy due to the bulkiness and filling high fibre content in fruit) to jeopardise your weight loss.

A note about appetite: it takes twenty minutes for your brain to register that you are satisfied, so eating quickly will mean you eat more than you need to feel full and you end up feeling bloated. You should feel satisfied but not uncomfortable or bloated; you should still be able to get up and move around with ease, and you should still be able to do your trousers up! The stomach is a muscle that can expand and contract, stretch and shrink back to its normal size (you can't make it any smaller than your natural size without surgery). You can train your stomach to be satisfied with smaller portions in a matter of days. Eat less than you normally would at the first few meals and you may feel like there is some room left, but as your stomach and brain adjust you will notice that smaller quantities are actually enough to leave you satisfied. As soon as you absentmindedly eat a meal of your previous sized larger plateful, you will be surprised at how stuffed you feel now that your stomach has got used to smaller quantities of food. But you still need to listen to your body and there will be some days when you are very active that you will naturally feel much more hungry, but these will be balanced by the not so active days when you don't feel like eating so much. As long as you listen to your body, everything will balance out.

Don't forget the odd treat though, as missing out on everything you love is not what life is about. Whilst you may not exactly need chocolate or other less healthy foods, allowing yourself the occasional small treat will stop you craving them. We could all eat perfectly all of the time, but wouldn't that be boring?

17 Conclusion

I hope I have shown you how it is possible to eat exactly what you want, just in the right proportions, and remain as healthy and slim as you wish. I never feel I am missing out because I never do – if I want to eat I will, even if it is something 'naughty' I'll have just a small amount.

Sometimes you will encounter mental battles – the desire for taste and gluttony is inevitable, and perfectly normal. After all some things just look too good not to eat! But the key is to balance foods in your overall diet, or to put it another way that old saying 'everything in moderation'. If you have a setback don't worry, just get back to eating normally straight away and no damage will be done. Sometimes you may feel tempted by what you know is ultimately unhelpful – a second or third slice of cake, another high calorie snack not long before a meal, that last big slice of pizza. Stop and think to yourself, 'do I need it?', 'do I really want it?' Can you balance it against what you eat the rest of the time? Is it worth having to exercise more or cut back on your food intake later? Would just a mouthful do instead?

I have talked about the pitfalls of deprivation numerous times throughout this book and how it actually only leads to craving these foods more. Now I want to point out how, as much as it is important to be fit and healthy and as much as everyone wants to look their best, this is only a very tiny aspect of life. You are a not just a physical being but a person with a character and a life, a job or place of study or a family to look after. You should have friends, interests, memories from the past and great things to look forward to in the future.

I wrote this book because I was frustrated at seeing so many people wasting so much time and energy, having their every waking moment dedicated to losing weight. This just isn't what life is about. I want to help people get back to eating normally and to free them from a pointless existence that revolves around trying with every drop of futile willpower not to eat. We need to eat! There's no getting around this fact so we might as well enjoy it as well as aiming to feel healthy and look good.

Either way, the choice is yours and how you look and feel is in your hands. Dieticians, personal trainers and self help gurus have been saying this for years. Now I hope what I have shown you is that you can do it without ever feeling hungry, never depriving yourself of any food, never buying expensive diet products or following a particular regime. You can be both slim and healthy and love your food. You just have to eat normally.

18 Troubleshooting

I want to lose weight sensibly by simply eating better, how do I get started?

Just start now! Or at the next meal or snack at least. If you put it off you may never get round to it or start to dread a looming 'D-Day', which will put you in a negative frame of mind. Why put it off any longer? If you've already started cooking your next meal and you think it may be quite high calorie, just eat less. Have some extra salad, vegetables or fruit if you are still hungry afterwards. See the ideas in *Chapter 7, Where Do I Go From Here* for when you next go food shopping. When you've finished reading this book you will probably know exactly what you need to do. There's no time like the present!

I've cut down my food and drink calories, why have I not lost weight?

How long ago did you start cutting down? Things won't happen overnight. Weigh yourself no more than once a week and on the same scales, first thing in the morning before eating or drinking, in light clothing such as nightwear or underwear. Our bodies fluctuate in weight every day due to water retention, bowel movements, menstrual cycles in women and even the volume (not the same as calorific value) of what we have eaten and drunk in the last 24 hours. See *Chapter 5, Where Are You Going Wrong?*, to check you are cutting down as much as you think you are. It is important to strike a balance between cutting down enough to lose weight, but not too much so that your metabolism slows down and you don't burn as much energy.

I'm exercising a lot, why have I not lost weight?

Weight loss only comes with burning more calories than you consume, so perhaps you are not burning off as much as you think. Cardiovascular exercises that get you out of breath are good for burning calories in the short term, but a healthy metabolism is supported by good muscle tone, so do some resistance or weight training too, if you can. If you are finding that exercise makes you hungrier you may actually be eating more; keeping a food diary should help you notice where the calories are coming from. Muscle weighs more than fat, so if you are building or toning muscles as you exercise you may even weigh more at first even if you haven't got 'bigger'. The plus side is that the extra muscle speeds up your metabolism so you will burn calories faster. Try monitoring your progress by measuring around your waist, thighs, upper arms and buttocks once a fortnight, and take note of how your clothes fit.

How do I lose weight from my tummy and arms but not my legs or bum?

Unfortunately how we are built is determined in our genetic make-up, and we can't change this. Cutting calories will make you lose weight, but you cannot change where this weight naturally comes off. What you can do, however, is to exercise the relevant areas to tone up the individual muscle groups, resulting in a more sculpted and proportioned figure. Tricep dips are good for upper arms, sit-ups for the stomach area, and squats for thighs and buttocks. A one-off session with a personal trainer or gym instructor should give you all the information you need on which exercises are best, or follow a DVD or join a class devised for body toning and sculpting.

I was doing really well and lost weight, but now I'm not losing any more weight even though I haven't changed anything.

The more you have to lose the faster your metabolism will be as you carry around all that extra weight. This means that the more weight you lose, the smaller your calorie requirements, and you may need to cut your calorie intake further or do more cardiovascular exercise to burn calories. Another way to keep your metabolism fast is to split you daily food intake into smaller meals, going for no longer than three hours between eating during the day, and do some resistance or strength exercises (see *Chapter 8, Exercise*), which increase the amount of muscle you have, and in turn make you burn fat at a faster rate even when you are resting.

I'm fed up of cooking separate meals for myself and my family, as I'm the only one on a diet.

Why are you cooking separate meals? If the food you give your family is so bad maybe they shouldn't be eating it either! You can eat the same as everyone else, just eat smaller portions and fill the rest of your plate with salad or vegetables. Alternatively why not give some of your family's favourite meals a health makeover; see *Chapter 12, Home Cooking Tricks*, for how to do this, or try some of the recipes I have provided. They are tasty and satisfying enough for everyone to enjoy, and calories are given for portions so you know what you are eating, though not everyone has to stick to the recommended portions if they have bigger calorie needs. Normal eating of normal foods, in amounts that don't exceed your needs, is the only method needed to be healthy and slim.

I've reached my goal weight. Now what?

Congratulations! You must be feeling really proud, not to mention having more energy and looking and feeling great. Now all you have to do is continue to eat what you have been eating most recently (in the past two to four weeks). Your weight should naturally plateau, due to your metabolism adjusting to your new weight and calorie intake, and remain stable. If you continue to lose weight then increase your calorie intake slightly, and if you ever gain weight again then follow the same steps you took to lose it. Whatever you do don't return to the way of eating that made you overweight in the first place. Now I think it's time for that well deserved shopping trip for some smaller clothes!

19 Diets are a Joke

Just for a bit of fun and because, let's face it, diets *are* a joke.

It isn't what you eat between Christmas and New Year; it's what you eat between New Year and Christmas.

Cosgrove

In the Middle Ages, they had guillotines, stretch racks, whips and chains. Nowadays, we have a much more effective torture device called the bathroom scales.

Stephen Phillips

I've been on a diet for two weeks and all I've lost is fourteen days.

Totie Fields

The word aerobics came about when the gym instructors got together and said, 'If we're going to charge £10 an hour, we can't call it jumping up and down.'

Rita Rudner

Food is like sex: when you abstain, even the worst stuff begins to look good.

Beth McCollister

I have gained and lost the same ten pounds so many times over and over again my cellulite must have déjà vu.

Jane Wagner

I lied on my support group food diary. I put down that I had three eggs... but they were chocolate cream eggs.

Caroline Rhea

My doctor told me to stop having intimate dinners for four. Unless there are three other people.

Orson Welles

I told my doctor I get very tired when I go on a diet, so he gave me pep pills. Know what happened? I ate faster.

Joe E. Lewis

The biggest seller is cookbooks and the second is diet books – how not to eat what you've just learned how to cook.

Andy Roone

References and Credits

1. www.bhf.org.uk
2. www.netdoctor.co.uk
3. www.bupa.co.uk
4. Shahrad Taheri, Ling Lin, Diane Austin, Terry Young and Emmanuel Mignot. 'Short Sleep Duration Is Associated with Reduced Leptin, Elevated Ghrelin, and Increased Body Mass Index', Public Library of Science. Medecine Journal. 2004 December;1(3):e62.
5. www.bmj.com
6. www.childgrowthfoundation.org
7. www.zonediet.com
8. www.weightwatchers.co.uk
9. www.grapefruitdiet.org
10. Health Via Food, Dr William Howard Hay M. D., 1932, Sun-Diet Health Service Inc.
11. www.therawfoodmovement.com
12. www.weightlossresources.co.uk
13. www.thefreedictionary.com/salad
14. www.drinkaware.co.uk
15. www.drinking.nhs.co.uk
16. www.dh.gov.uk
17. www.walkingspree.com
18. www.nhs.uk
19. www.quotegarden.com
20. www.eatwell.gov.uk and www.food.gov.uk, www.nhs.uk/Livewell/Goodfood/Pages/eight-tips-healthy-eating.aspx
21. www.caloriecount.about.com
22. www.nutrition.org.uk
23. Chichester Nutrition & Dietics Department, St Richard's Hospital, 2006
24. www.quorn.co.uk
25. www.thedietplate.com; trial registration at clinicaltrials.gov [3], identifier: NCT00254124_Arch Intern Med. 2007;167:1277-1283_
26. www.shakspeareeditorial.co.uk
27. Baby-led Weaning, Gill Rapley and Tracey Murkett, 2008, Ebury Publishing

Credits

All photographs in *Eat, Drink and be Slim* (unless otherwise indicated) are the copyrighted property of **123RF Limited**, their Contributors or Licensed Partners and are being used with permission under license. These images and/or photos may not be copied or downloaded without permission from 123RF Limited.

'H' Photography (Cover photo) – www.hphotography.co.uk

Barbara James (Editor) – barbara.james5@btopenworld.com

Alison Shakspeare (Design) – www.shakspeareeditorial.or

About the Author

London born Polly first studied nutrition whilst training to be a dancer in her late teens and early twenties. A healthy diet plays an important role in keeping in peak condition for dancers, but unlike other sports where performance is the focus, dancers are pressured to be slim and physically attractive to get work too, and this can drive young dancers to all sorts of unhealthy methods in attempts to lose weight quickly for auditions. Polly picked up many tips, both healthy and unhealthy, along the way, but can now use that knowledge to make informed choices about how and what to eat to stay both slim AND healthy.

Nutrition as a subject was covered more comprehensively whilst studying for an HND in Beauty and Health Therapy Management at Chichester College, equipping Polly with detailed knowledge of how food impacts health and wellbeing as well as weight.

Polly acquired the qualification of Metabolic Effect Nutrition Consultant, and followed this by co-founding and becoming a director of The Fit Mum Formula, who provide online nutritional and fitness programmes in a more detailed and comprehensive way, focusing on fat loss, and increased muscle tone, leading to a more effective metabolism and addressing issues such as insulin resistance and the effects different foods have on your hormonal disposition.

These days Polly has a creditably healthy attitude towards food. This, combined with her knowledge of nutrition, enables her to be both slim and healthy whilst enjoying any food she likes in a normal, sociable, realistic way, enjoying the odd burger or piece of cake as much as the rest of us.

Polly is a full-time Mum to four-year-old Aurora and one-year-old Bella, whom she wants to have a healthy, relaxed attitude towards food in a world where even children are being inundated with images of 'perfect' bodies and complex dietary advice. She decided to write this book out of frustration at the ridiculous diet advice and claims we are frequently bombarded with by the media, who cash in on our insecurities and weight problems with their impressively creative nonsense which serves only to not work, so that readers will buy the next publication looking for an alternative solution. Two thirds of UK adults are overweight, and it has been suggested that if trends continue 25 percent of children will be obese by 2050[1]. With Polly having witnessed first-hand the effects of yo-yo dieting and unhealthy weightloss methods as a dancer, the importance of staying healthy is something she feels very passionate about. Not only for herself but also to set a new positive health forecast for future generations.

www.ingramcontent.com/pod-product-compliance
Lightning Source LLC
Chambersburg PA
CBHW041259040426
42334CB00028BA/3089